THE SYNORGON DIET
How To Achieve Healthy Weight In A World Of Excess

by
Dr. R. L. Wysong

Inquiry Press

The information contained in this book has been compiled for purposes of education. The views and conclusions expressed by the author and cited sources do not represent all-inclusive knowledge or unanimity of opinion, and should not be construed as specific medical advice.

First Edition

Published by Inquiry Press
1880 North Eastman, Midland, Michigan 48640

Printed in the United States of America

ISBN 0-918112-06-0

About the cover

 The continuous links interlocked around the Synorgon "S", symbolize the inextricable connection between all living and inanimate elements in our universe. The display of the Synorgon logo is to remind us of our interconnection with the environment.

To those for whom life
has greater responsibility
than living

CONTENTS

Figures .... *iv*

Synorgon Defined .... *ix*

Foreword .... *x*

Introduction .... *xvi*

Section I - What You Need To Know

1 - Synorgon Rationale 1

2 - The Scope of the Problem 10

3 - The Miracle of Weight Maintenance 15

4 - Our Genetic Roots.................................... 20

5 - Obesity's Environmental Toll.................... 29

6 - Obesity's Health Toll 38

7 - Measuring Fat.. 48

8 - Lipids 51

9 - A Calorie Is Not A Calorie 57

10 - Genetics 70

11 - Food As An Addiction 75

12 - Food & Mood 89

13 - Appetite 96

14 - Exercise 102

15 - Fiber 111

16 - The Obese Personality 115

17 - Gain & Loss 125

18 - Autoimmunity..132

19 - Obesity In The Young.............................137

20 - Too Much of Too Little...........................141

21 - Good Fats, Bad Fats 153

22 - Interventions 162

Table Of Contents

Section II- What You Need To Do

23 - Guidelines Introduction 173

24 - Eat For Health, Not For Weight 176

25 - Change Should Be Gradual 177

26 - Get Smart; Use Foresight 181

27 - Balance Sympathetic
     And Parasympathetic Activities 183

28 - Seek Healthy Companions 184

29 - Make Exercise A Part Of Everyday Life 185

30 - Take Time To Eat 190

31 - Change The Number Or Size Of Meals 192

32 - Simplify Meals 195

33 - Eat Portions And Leave Some 197

34 - Emphasize Complex Carbohydrates 198

35 - Reduce Flavors 200

36 - Convert To Whole, Fresh, Raw Foods 202

37 - Seek Foods Rich In Natural Micronutrients 204

38 - Choose Only Packaged Foods
     Which Are Low In Fat 205

39 - Consume Optimal Trace Minerals And Vitamins ... 207

40 - Rich, Natural Sources Of Omega -3
     Fatty Acids Should Be Increased 208

41 - Restore The Environment 210

42 - Lose Without Dieting 211

43 - Crutches 214

44 - Diet For One Day 218

45 - Conclusion 220

Appendixes

I - Lipid Biochemistry 223
    Fatty Acids 223
    Nomenclature...226
    Phospholipids...226
    Isomers 229
    Biological Membranes 231
II - Lipid Digestion 237
III - Adipose Tissue 242
IV - Companion Animal Recommendations 248

More Resources by Dr. Wysong.....................................258
Index 264

FIGURES

Foreward

F-1   Technology and Industrialization .... *viii*

Chapters

1 - Synorgon Rationale

1-1   Without A Roadmap........................... 1

1-2   Time-line Chart (200 year) 3

1-3   Is Decreasing Mortality Due To
Modern Technology.......................... 5

1-4   Synergy 8

3 - The Miracle Of Weight Maintainance

3-1   Just One Bite 16

3-2   Eat All of the Four Food Groups 18

4 - Our Genetic Roots

4-1   Fat World = Fat Us 20

4-2   Cavemen - In The Wild.................... 21

4-3   Over the Oily River 22

4-4   Honk If You Love Mother Earth 23

4-5   Timeline - Rate of Change
In the Last 200 Years...................... 23

4-6   Genetic Expectations 24

4-7   The Grand Experiment 25

4-8   Fish Out Of Water 26

4-9   The Influence of Modern Society 27

5 - Obesity's Environmental Toll

5-1   Chicken/Cow/Pig Man 30

5-2   Golden Arches 31

5-3   Wheaners 31

5-4   Care For Some Freshly Ground Beef 32

5-5   What Can I Get For You (Meat Counter) 34

5-6   Suicide of a Vegetarian 36

6 - Obesity's Health Toll
    6-1   Standmill, Televisercise, Bicep Curls & Airobics .. 43
    6-2   The Obesity Pain Reflex 45

7 - Measuring Fat
    7-1   Height and Weight Table 49

8 - Lipids
    8-1   Stay Away From Fatty Acids 52
    8-2   Functions Of Fatty Acids 54

9 - A Calorie Is Not A Calorie
    9-1   Sun Energy 58
    9-2   Food Type Efficiency 62

10 - Genetics
    10-1   The Obesity Gene 73

11 - Food As An Addiction
    11-1   Healthy Balance 78
    11-2   Unhealthy Imbalance...................................... 79
    11-3   Mmmm...Feels Good 81
    11-4   Some Neurotransmitters, Their Functions
            and The Nutrient Precursors........................... 83
    11-5   Disgusted 86
    11-6   Beautiful Day 87

12 - Food & Mood
    12-1   Carbohydrates and Mood.............................. 90
    12-2   Climb Walls 92
    12-3   Reducing Salon 93
    12-4   Glycemic Index 94

13 - Appetite
    13-1   Bob's Body Was a Temple 98
    13-2   "On" Eating Switch 100

14 - Exercise
   14-1   Don's Salon 103
   14-2   Pump Food System 105
   14-3   Never Used 108

15 - Fiber
   15-1   Granny Fiber 112
   15-2   If You Want Extra Fiber 113

16 - Attitude
   16-1   The Eye-Mouth Gap... 118
   16-2   Don't Ever Give Up 120
   16-3   The Ups And Downs On The Road
          To Weight Success 121

17 - Gain & Loss
   17-1   The Results Of Repeated Gain And Loss........... 126
   17-2   Better Not To Have Dieted
          Than To Diet And Regain 128

18 - Autoimmunity
   18-1   Immune Dysfunction 135

19 - Obesity In The Young
   19-1   How Obesity Begins 137
   19-2   Sloth Hybrid 138
   19-3   Child Coax 139

20 - Too Much Of Too Little
   20-1   Food Sources And Processing Losses 145
   20-2   Comparison Of Domestic
          and Wild Animal Meat..................................... 146
   20-3   The Rise of Food Color 149
   20-4   The Rise of Soft Drinks 149
   20-5   Fresh Fruit vs. Processed Fruit 149
   20-6   The Rise of Sweeteners 149
   20-7   Confusing The System 150

21 - Good Fats, Bad Fats

21-1   Processing Alterations 155

21-2   Lipid Oxidation 156

21-3   Free Radical Damage To Membranes 157

21-4   The Formation of Atheroma 159

22 - Interventions

22-1   Jejunotransverse Colostomy 164

22-2   Gastric Bypass 165

22-3   Vertical Banded Gastroplasty.......................... 166

22-4   Lady in Front of Medical Center 167

22-5   Typical Diet Drink Ingredient List 170

25 - Change Should Be Gradual

25-1   Rate of Weight Loss For Obese Patients 180

29 - Make Exercise A Part Of Everyday Life

29-1   Ad About Tying Shoes 187

30 - Take Time To Eat

30-1   Don't Eat Like This 190

31 - Change The Number Or Size Of Meals

31-1   Pancreatic Size 192

38 - Choose Only Packaged Foods Which Are Low In Fat

38-1   Fat Free Water 205

42 - Lose Without Dieting

42-1   Lose - No Diet 212

42-2   A Bad Buy 213

Appendixes

I - Lipid Biochemistry

I-1   Fatty Acid Structure 223

I-2   Structure Of A Triglyceride 224

I-3   Linoleic And Linolenic Acid
        Structure & Nomenclature.............................225

I-4   Nomenclature And Structure
        Of Common Fatty Acids 226

I-5   Structure Of Phospholipids.............................229

I-6   Isomers 230

I-7   Fatty Acid Configurations 231

I-8   Membrane Lipids 232

I-9   Triglyceride Fluidity 233

I-10   Bilipid Cell Membrane 235

II - Lipid Digestion

II-1   Micelle Transport...238

II-2   Lipid Absorption Chart 239

III - Adipose Tissue

III-1   Triacylglycerols 245

III-2   The Chain Maintaining Normal Weight............246

IV - Companion Animal Recommendations

IV-1   Pets And Owners Look Alike 249

IV-2   Doctor, Mother, Child & Pet 250

IV-3   Chicken May Not Be Chicken...........................253

IV-4   The Dangerous Middle 254

IV-5   I Feel So Much Healthier..................................255

IV-6   Everyone Should Join A Health Club 256

SYNORGON DEFINED

[1]In an attempt to describe our place in the universe and its relationship to health, I have found existing terminology insufficient or presently inappropriate. *Holism, vitalism, naturalism, Gaiaism* and like terms touch aspects of the concept, but seem either too narrow or have become distorted over time by popular misinterpretation or prejudice. For example, *natural* may conjure up images of a "natural" fruit juice containing only 5% fruit juice; *vitalism* is viewed as refuse cast aside by the scientific, mechanistic era; and *holism* might smack of snake venom, crystal therapy or other supposedly quackish medical practices. In other words, words have failed me, so I've created a new one. *Synorgon* is new and fresh, which relieves me of having to defend a particular definition of someone else's word or struggle to redefine it, and permits me to make a word what I want it to be without argument.

Weight control, health, and environmental problems need a fresh and more fundamental approach. What better way to begin than with a new word...synorgon.

syn-or-gon[1] (sin´ôr-gon) *n.* [*synergy* interrelatedness, co-operation + *organism* life, complexity] **1.** the larger interconnected thing of which everything is a part. **2.** the universe resulting from the interrelatedness of all cosmic things known, unknown, understood, not comprehended and incomprehensible. **3.** all of existence as a dynamic, interconnected, cooperative, synergetic, balanced living organism of which we are simply a part. **4.** our entire physical and biological greater context as if it were essential to our existence and health. **5.** all of existence, the parts of which are seen to be on a continuum with all other parts, the qualities of which are emergent and unpredicted by the reductionistic analysis of the parts. **6.** all of existence as it functions without artificial manipulation: Unmanipulated, it is healthy; manipulated, such that balances and interconnections are disrupted, it is diseased. — **synorgon´ic,** *adj.* — **synorgonis´tic,** *adj.* —**synor´gonous,** *adv.* of the nature of synorgon —**syn´orgon´omy,** *n.* the study of synorgon —**synor´gonism,** *n.* a deduction or principle derived from synorgonomy —**mi´crosyn´orgon,** *n.* a smaller entity reflecting in a limited sense synorgonic principles — **mac´rosyn´orgon,** *n.* a larger composite of microsynorgons.

All things have a price. The safety, security, convenience, luxury, and ease of the industrial/technological era are all at a cost. This cost is, of course, in part monetary because we all must pay for the goods of modern life. But this is only a partial payment, and a discount at that. No one is paying the full price for the massive disruption of our Earth and its resources.

Most of us feel that we work hard for a living. This may be true, but the living we get is often disproportionate to the work we do. One middle-income person's wage from a mere forty hours of work per week might feed and clothe a family of five, and over time provide a 2,000-square-foot home, a vacation cabin, furnishings, two cars, a recreational vehicle, snowmobile, insurance to replace it all if lost, taxes to support public services, bureaucracy, social aid, defense, and part of a 800 billion dollar per year medical industry, plus enough to college educate three children, allow some dabbling in the stock market, and generate revenues for retirement by age 55.

The modern ability to harvest the resources of the Earth at an incredible pace enables us to live at bargain prices. Compare what once was done by axe to the present ability to harvest and mill acres of timber in a single day. Compare farming by hand to that possible in today's industrialized agriculture.

It would appear that with modern technology we get more than we earn. We do. If so, who or what is making up the difference?

It is the Earth itself and its resources which are being reaped in excess of the price paid. What is the proper price? Whatever is necessary to assure the sustenance of the resources for use by future generations. $1.39 is not the correct price for an eight-foot 2 x 4 board, unless that price also covers the cost to renew the forest from which it came, to clean pollutants which may have resulted from its milling, and to replace the energy required for its production and transportation with a clean, renewable source.

Not only is modern voluptuary living a tremendous bargain but it also shifts much of the costs of its indulgences to future generations. It is as if we mine the Earth, put it through a factory to produce our products of leisure, and directly hook the chimneys and effluent pipes into a future generation. We are cheating: not only do we steal and play with the toys of our children, but after playing, we leave the mess for them to clean up. The environmental price is therefore another part of the equation which we are not paying.

We have not, however, been able to steal without being caught or to totally seal the exhaust pipes diverting environmental damage into our children's generation. Some is leaking out. We are now beginning to suffer some of the consequences of our myopic excesses. Acid rain, oil spills, Chernobyls, Love Canals and Bhoepal represent only headlined tips of the iceberg. Consider also the following problems. While less easily recognized, these are also parts of the treacherous iceberg:

- Soil erosions from treating living soil as if it were a strip mine
- Toxicants used on crops to increase yields
- Ever-lower micronutrient levels in food crops harvested year after year with only NPK (nitrogen, phosphorous, potassium) fertilizer used to replace nutrients lost
- Food processing designed to increase profits by increasing shelf life and flavor rather than nutrient value
- An ever-increasing demand for and supply of sybaritic products of ease, many of which are unnecessary.
  Does each of us really need three cars, 20 pairs of shoes,

a garbage disposal, air conditioner, six suits, 30 ties, three
TVs, 200 toys or 60 bottles of cosmetics? (It is likely that
less than one percent of purchases from modern multi-acre
shopping malls, often built over natural habitat, are for
true necessities.)
* A growing dependence on professionals and loss of self-
sufficiency
* An ever-increasing disengagement from the Earth, our
natural heritage, as we become more and more insulated
from it by "things" and "stuff"

Life in a synthetic world confuses our origins and responsibilities. If the Earth were infinite or if this generation were
the only one to which an ethic need be applied, then our
present course of plundering the Earth's resources would be
proper and right. But neither is the case. The Earth's reserves
are finite, and morally it can be argued that this generation has
no right to steal and squander the sustenance required for, or
the natural beauty desired by, the next generation. Pretending
that we are separate and apart from nature and that we can
squander its riches is a deadly mistake. The ultimate consequence of such imbalance is the loss of health.

Now what does all this have to do with maintaining healthy
weight? Simply that the bloat of obesity is a part of the bloat
of society at large. We're fat in our home, closet, garage, car,
office — just about everywhere you look. Why would we not be
fat on our bodies? If modern technology did not present the
option for excesses both in food and leisure, if it did not permit
the dramatic alteration of our environment and the character
of our food supply, if the only food available were that picked
raw, fresh, and whole, directly from nature, and we had to
expend considerable effort to find and harvest it, then obesity
would not exist. Nor would many other degenerative, environmentally induced or influenced illnesses.

That's a lot of ifs, and some big ones at that. The idea of
each of us now skipping through the bushes in our loincloths

each day collecting berries falls far short of practical possibility. Much of modern technology was, in fact, designed to feed and protect from the elements, a swelling population. What would we do now, for example, without modern sanitation, utilities or food distribution? Disease would abound and starvation decimate the population. We are now faced with the apparent dilemma of being able to live neither with modern technology nor without it.

But technology and industrialization have taken us far beyond assisting us to survive, into the world of frills and excess. A perfect example is the automobile. That which would be necessary for transportation, comfort, safety and energy efficiency is entirely unlike the chromed, gas-guzzling death traps which have flooded the highways for the past decades and undergone an unnecessary aesthetic model change every year. Practical solutions to living problems have become lost in the excitement of the marketing opportunities and profits made possible by technological capabilities.

Technology, like any tool, has the capacity for good or bad. It is one thing to use technology to solve problems of transportation, food production and distribution, housing, clothing, and so forth, while at the same time preventing waste, pollu-

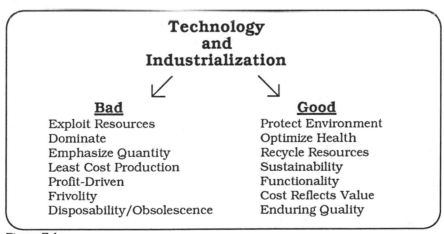

Figure F-1

tion or health consequences. It is quite another thing to create overabundance or frivolous new gadgets, simply to produce profit and inflated wages (excesses which in turn fuel additional consumption and further motivate profiteers in an endless spiral).

It is mind that has brought us the incredible ability to alter our environment and manipulate its resources. It is mind which must reorientate our actions to the benefit of this and future generations. The grocery cart has replaced the spear. The cunning necessary for sorting through food, consumer products, and lifestyle choices replaces the cunning required to survive in the wild.

If we allow ourselves simply to be swept along by the flow of money, not by a broad ethic or fiduciary responsibility, consequences will result. Obesity is merely one consequence befalling some of us. Others fall victim to stress-related diseases, environmental illnesses, occupational diseases, and a host of arguably nutrition-related degenerative diseases such as heart and vascular disease, cancer, arthritis, senility, adult onset diabetes, and autoimmunities — all to a large extent a result of a society targeting excessive profits rather than health and sustainability.

Solving problems of weight, therefore, becomes a matter of taking control and making choices, not simply being led by others who may not have your best interests in mind. Purchasing and using everything that we are urged to buy on a billboard or TV commercial is a certain road to disaster.

Choices must be made. If those choices are within the synorgonic backdrop of understanding our natural heritage and the need to restore balances, then lasting progress is possible.

Weight control approached with these understandings will not only bring the many benefits of increased individual health, but also raise our consciousness about larger issues of social and environmental responsibility. It will be through such individual awareness, action, and pressure on society's policy-makers that our world can progress toward the paradisaic health and peace it is possible to achieve.

———————

INTRODUCTION

The accumulation of excess body fat is a problem of epidemic proportions among developed societies. The insidious results rob people of health, shorten life, adversely affect the environment, and make pleasurable and full living difficult, if not, in some cases, impossible to achieve. Although weight management has become commonplace and practically a way of life for millions, the consequences of the condition, the complexity of its causes, and its relationship to our larger universe context — the synorgon — are little understood and appreciated.

Excess weight is viewed as a profit opportunity for salons and product manufacturers, and yet another buying "necessity" for consumers, rather than a serious and real social and physiological disease requiring understanding and fundamental changes. Ours is an overfed society seeking immediate palliation and cures rather than rational long-term approaches to prevention and health enhancement. When we have a problem, we tend to look for a remedy that is simple — something easy, cheap, and fast. Though they may seem appealing, a special "magic in a bottle," a pill, an easy exercise, exotic food, or clever surgery invariably misses the mark. Life, by nature, is more complex than anyone can even begin to imagine. The distortion of life, which is what excess weight is, is therefore likewise complex. Solutions similarly must address complexity. They must be as big as the problem. It is futile and naive to hope to solve complex health issues with silver bullet solutions.

Fortunately, while the physiological, environmental, and social factors causing obesity are complex, the synorgonic solutions, although often difficult to implement, are based on a concept easy to understand and at least intuitively known by nearly everyone. That concept is, quite simply, that *we have extracted ourselves from our natural synorgonic environmental roots. If we are out of our proper context, then returning to it is the solution.* This understanding provides a philosophic paradigm for healthy weight maintenance, as well as a more effective approach both to health care in general, and also to environmental health.

This book is designed to convince you of this simple truth. Only when this is accomplished and the meaning of this concept is inextricably implanted into the will and applied in daily living, can the lasting changes occur which are essential to maintaining healthy weight.

There are three general divisions in the book. The first section — "What You Need To Know" — will help you understand the mechanisms at work in our bodies and in our environment that lead to weight maintenance problems. Although a little technical at times, this section will broaden and deepen your understanding so that effective, life-long changes can be made. Although everyone wants quick, bottom-line answers to fix their weight problem, a quick, easy-fix approach simply does not work to achieve lasting healthy weight. Our minds have created a world and a lifestyle that in turn creates disease, including obesity; our minds must be used to correct the dilemma.

The second section — "What You Need To Do" — gets into the specifics. Here you will learn how to put into action in everyday life the principles you have learned in the first section of the book. Although pointing to specific remedies, this section is certainly not all-inclusive. It need not be, since the real value of the Synorgon Diet is that you will learn to be able to make your own healthy life, healthy weight choices.

The last section is a series of appendixes. The topics in the appendixes are technically in depth. Everyone should at least skim these chapters when it is suggested to do so in the first two sections of the book. Those more techni- cally skilled will benefit by reading them carefully to more fully grasp the biology of weight maintenance. The last appendix ap- plies the principles discussed throughout the book to caring for companion animals, in seeking to prevent and reverse weight prob- lems that have become epidemic for them as well.

————————

Section I

What You Need
To Know

1 - SYNORGON RATIONALE

Good health requires a good underlying philosophy

If you tried to reach Miami from Chicago without road signs or a map, would you expect to get there? Even if you drove the speed limit, used your directional signals and changed the oil, it would be unlikely. Although driving rules are important, and they may keep you safe and your car running, they don't get you there.

Similarly, if your destination is good health and normal weight, you need a guide, a philosophy — a road map. Simply counting calories, measuring protein and fat, chewing each bite twenty times or doing thirty sit-ups a day doesn't get you there. Such "rules" may help, be a good part of an overall program and keep you running, but they won't get you to your destination — lasting results.

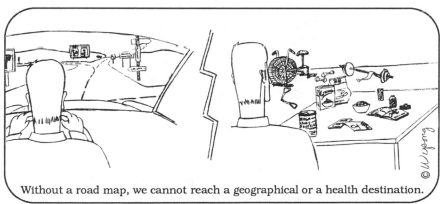

Without a road map, we cannot reach a geographical or a health destination.

Figure 1-1

This book is designed to give guidance, to convince you of a reasonable philosophy, to provide a road map rather than to simply enumerate rules.

The logic for the Synorgon Diet surpasses that of any other competing idea. If I can convince you of the synorgonic principle, then you will have a useful filter through which information can be sorted and choices made. You will have the road map to a life of healthy weight. This book thus provides the key to a new life for you based on knowledge and control.

But first let me show you why the very thing (information) which should solve our problems (including weight control) does not.

The synorgonic philosophy filters out erroneous health concepts

We live in an age of mushrooming knowledge. The plethora of competing ideas, diet plans, and products designed to relieve obesity is but one example of confusion in part created by the sheer mass of information available to us.

The glut of data is bewildering and confusing without sound philosophic concepts against which this information can resonate. Good health, good medicine, does not simply mean the implementation of the latest technology. It begins with philosophy.

As Galen, a second century physician, argued — "the best physician is also a philosopher." But few physicians today are. They too fall victim to dazzling technology. Starry-eyed, they are led by it rather than led by a carefully thought through life philosophy. So don't feel alone if you're confused and do not know for sure which way to turn. Even the "experts" are fumbling along.

The information age does not equal the truth age

You see — increasing information does not necessarily mean increasing truth. Although discovery and knowledge are growing, facts often become distorted as they are used to support or advance some cherished idea. Given the same body of evidence, there exist hundreds of competing interpretations in religion, politics, history, medicine, and science. Yet, each argues that they are supported by the facts. Resistance

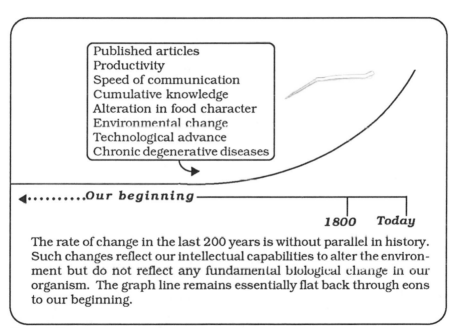

Published articles
Productivity
Speed of communication
Cumulative knowledge
Alteration in food character
Environmental change
Technological advance
Chronic degenerative diseases

◄·········*Our beginning*

1800 *Today*

The rate of change in the last 200 years is without parallel in history. Such changes reflect our intellectual capabilities to alter the environment but do not reflect any fundamental biological change in our organism. The graph line remains essentially flat back through eons to our beginning.

Figure 1-2

to change, preconceptions (if it's what I've been taught, then it must be true), economic advantage, and desire for power cause facts to be both distorted and selected.

Thus, the mere explosion of information does not necessarily bring us closer to truth.

Facts as raw pieces of data, regardless of their quantity, are meaningless. They must be interpreted to mold new or support old ideas.

Unfortunately, newness — or change — is uncomfortable for most minds. Prejudice, tradition, vested interest, and ego all tend to force data into pre-existing molds. Society is not led by a zeal for truth but rather by powerful economic and socio-political forces bent on maintaining status quo. Those in power want to remain there and those economically comfortable want to remain so. The sheer inertia of a belief system can hold it in place for centuries, even if it is wrong.

Beliefs are often held for reasons other than rationalism

History is, in fact, simply a junkyard of discarded "truths," "truths" that held minds captive for centuries, even millenia, and for which the blood of millions has been spilled.

Economic, political, egocentric truth-molding forces are at work with vigor even in science and medicine. For example, in medicine, centuries after facts were available that contradicted them, wrong ideas were maintained. Examples include blood letting and septic surgical techniques which have only relatively recently been rejected.

Lest we be led to believe that now modern medicine has everything all figured out or that they have a pill, diet or surgical procedure that could surely remedy our weight problems, let me continue.

**Modern
medicine
is bloated
with
retained
error**

The rise and fall of historical medical fallacies does not imply that modern health approaches, that our ideas here today, are the culmination of a battle for truth. Not so. Today, more than ever, ideas compete for money and power more than truth.

We need now be especially suspicious since modern medicine is not a family doctor making house calls, but a gigantic, highly profitable industrial complex. Modern health care is burdened with scientific fallacies propped up by selective data. It has become bloated with retained errors.

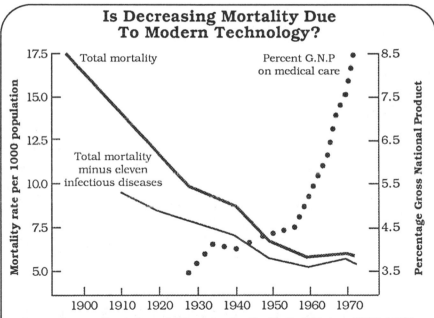

**Is Decreasing Mortality Due
To Modern Technology?**

Age and sex-adjusted mortality rates for the United States, 1900-1973. Including and excluding eleven major infectious diseases. Contrasted with the proportion of the Gross National Product expended on medical care. Notice how the drop in mortality is not related to the burgeoning cost of modern medical care. From "The Questionable Contribution of Medical Measures to the Decline of Mortality in the United States in the Twentieth Century" by John B. McKinlay and Sonja M. McKinlay.

Figure 1-3

Examples include the popular (professional and public) belief that early diagnosis is the same as prevention, that the allopathic (symptomatic) approach to medicine is the most effective, that modern technology and medicine have made us live longer, that we know what a 100 percent complete diet is, that synthetic fractionated foods are equal or superior to natural ones, that serious disease cannot be cured with nutritional and lifestyle modification, and that modern medical procedures have been proved by carefully controlled trials. All of these are commonly held modern fallacies.[1]

Irrationality is the square root of all evil

We must not confuse the technocratic age with true progress.[2]

Now where does all this discussion about information, truth, right, wrong, and bias lead us? Irrationality is the square root of all evil. If disease is an "evil," which it could certainly be argued to be, then it is likely the result of irrationality, or untruth. Obesity and other chronic or debilitating diseases are therefore a likely result of an untruth. That untruth and its damage to us (since we act upon what we believe), lies within our philosophic approach to health.

Our modern abundance of information has somehow been used to shore up wrong ideas. It therefore becomes necessary to back up, to reappraise our position to see if another approach better fits the facts.

As I said, it is possible to pick and choose data to support virtually any life choice. But if we are seeking solid and sound direction, something we can feel comfortable with and confident in for a lifetime, something as close to truth as we can find, a measure of effort must be put in up front to define one's philosophic position. This effort is well spent because it will prevent much wasted time — and perhaps harm — that can come from exploring all of the dead-end roads of ideas to which we are constantly exposed.

More time should be spent refining underlying broad philosophical ideas

So, if you will, put aside your preconceptions about weight control. Forget for the moment calorie counting, cholesterol, sit-ups, starving, self-denial, or the trust that an expert somewhere in our wonderful technological era has the easy answer all figured out for you.

Instead, listen to me — well at least for this book anyway. I will not give you yet another expert remedy. Instead I hope to guide you to what you already know. The solution to weight control is actually intuitive. It is smothered however by the barrage of commercialized solutions we are all exposed to.

Once this common sense intuitive understanding is unveiled in your mind, you will be able to develop a philosophy of weight control that is sound, solid, reasonable and yours.

The Synorgon Diet is simply an extrapolation of this logic you already possess. I call it the synorgon philosophy. That philosophy argues that we are part of an intricate web of

Synergy

All things interrelate. Food and Life are inter-
dependent, as are Earth-wide ecological rela-
tions and forces and laws within the universe
as a whole. Additionally, each of these systems
is interrelated with one another. Focusing on
parts rather than relationships will lead to
partial and erroneous conclusions.

Figure 1-4

*Seeing
our place
within
synorgon
is the key
to normal
weight and
health*

existence. If we live in harmony with that web,
we are more likely to benefit with health than
if we act in contradiction to it.

The synorgon philosophy argues that we
should eat foods as close to their natural
state as possible and live our lives as consis-
tently with our natural environmental context as possible. This is the take-away from
this book. If you are already convinced,
perhaps I can reinforce your belief and help
you implement it. If you are not, let me try to
persuade you.

1. Less than 20 percent of modern medical measures have been proved by controlled trials: "Assessing the Efficacy and Safety of Medical Technologies." U.S. Office of Technology Assessment for Publication, #PB286-929, p. 7.
2. Wysong, R.L. *Rationale for Nutrition*, Midland, MI: The Wysong Institute, 1990.

Most of us know if we have a battle of the bulge. Pants or skirts tighten, belts lengthen and we increasingly shop the "big and tall" or "plus sizes" departments. But we're not overweight — we're just a little hefty, pleasantly plump, large boned, nervous or just unable to lose after the last child. The mind is a wonderful thing.

Obesity is a serious disease, however, whether it is denied or not. The following criteria are more objective measures of whether you have a weight problem or not. Use the sobering results as the first step in a resolve to achieve and maintain healthy weight.

Obesity is defined as being 20 percent over normal weight

Obesity is defined as exceeding ideal body weight by 20 percent, or having a body mass index — weight in kilograms divided by height in meters — of 26 or more.[1] Morbid (very serious, life threatening) obesity is at least twice ideal weight, or 100 pounds over ideal weight.[2]

There are many classifications for the various types of obesity. Hyperplastic obesity describes the occurrence of an increased number of fat (adipose) cells, whereas the hyperophic type is characterized by increased fat-cell size. Android (central) obesity is typically an increase in abdominal fat girth, a condition most common in males. Gynoid (peripheral) obesity affects the lower body area — the hips and buttocks — and is more common in females. Obesity can occur in childhood or be adult-onset, and it can range in severity from mild to severe to morbid.[3]

Such technical language, however, has its dangers. If you are told you have morbid android hyperplastic obesity, it sounds like a disease over which you have little control, and one that surely requires medical intervention. It also gives the medical technocrat the illusion of knowledge and control. Neither is necessarily true. A quick glance at the American population clearly reveals that obesity is a rapidly growing problem of epidemic proportions. Obviously, in spite of advances in language, solutions are not prevailing.

90 percent of all Americans feel they are overweight

In 1987, 51 million Americans were overweight. In 1988 the number grew to 82 million. In 1974, 8.4 million adults were severly obese. By 1986 there were 14 million severely obese adults.[4] Obesity in females over 60 now exceeds 50 percent.[5] Obesity in children is likewise epidemic.[6]

There are ethnic and economic differences. Poor black women are twice as likely as affluent white women to be overweight, while the opposite is true of men. Thus, in American society, rich women tend to be thin and rich men overweight.[7]

Almost 90 percent of all Americans today feel they are overweight (whether they are or not), according to a 1985 Gallup poll. Consequently, more than 10 billion dollars are spent each year in an attempt to get slim.[8]

"Lite" products are now a 30 billion dollar per year business.[9] Nearly half of all normal-weight American women, and up to half of the U.S. adult population as a whole, are participants in weight loss programs.[10,11]

Interestingly, companion animals have come to mirror the very problems their masters have created for themselves. Human lifestyles and eating patterns have been forced upon these creatures. Obesity is the most common nutritional disease in dogs.[12] Forty percent of all dogs are believed to be overweight, as are 12 percent of all cats.[13] One study showed that there are almost twice as many obese dogs living with obese owners as obese dogs belonging to normal-weight owners.[14] Horses, pet birds, reptiles, camelids — virtually every creature taken in by humans and exposed to our way of life — becomes vulnerable to the same crippling disease. Obesity in millions of domesticated animals manifests itself in degenerative disease that taxes the animals, their owners and the veterinary care industry.

Animals often mirror the weight problems of their human caretakers

Since wild animals do not suffer from obesity, its appearance in domesticated animals is further proof of the thesis of this book — that weight imbalance is an artificially imposed problem resulting from disrupted synorgonic balance.

Given the scope of the problem, it might seem that we are biologically flawed. This is a convenient conclusion because it implies that it is not our fault that we are "broken." It is also a profitable conclusion, since broken things create the potential for a large service and repair industry, to provide products, professionals, diet centers, and written and video instructional guides.

Unfortunately, the problem is not a simple one of flawed or broken but easily repaired physiological mechanics. Neither is obesity simply a matter of weak character or lack of discipline. Setting aside rare genetic weaknesses, the blame in part goes to the Industrial Age, and in part to us who allow ourselves to be blindly led by it. Once we are hooked, powerful and addicting physiological processes become perverted, and then compel us to continue in our error.

Weight maintenance is an intricate, complex, and delicate balance that is wonderfully self-regulating unless we, through choice, abuse it or allow ourselves to be led too far out of our proper synorgonic context by the Industrial Age.

Part of my goal therefore will be to help you understand the complexity of the problem. This in turn will help prevent worthless and even dangerous digressions into simplistic (often dangerous) fad diet approaches.

---

1. Bouchard, Claude. "Is Weight Fluctuation a Risk Factor?" The New England Journal of Medicine 324 (1991): 1887.
2. Van Itallie, T. B., and Kral, J. G. "The Dilemma of Morbid Obesity." The Journal of The American Medical Association 246 (1981): 999-1003.
3. Schlundt, David G., et al. "A Behavioral Taxonomy of Obese Female Participants in a Weight-Loss Program."

The American Journal of Clinical Nutrition 53 (1991): 1151.

4. Council on Scientific Affairs, "Treatment of Obesity in Adults." The Journal of The American Medical Association 260 (1988): 2547.

5. "Ten-State Nutrition Survey," 1968-70, U.S. Dept. of Health, Education, and Welfare Publication No. (HSM) 72-8130, 1972. Atlanta, Centers for Disease Control.

6. Frankle, Reva T., and Yang, Mei-Uih. *Obesity and Weight Control.* Gaithersburg, Maryland: Aspen Publishers, Inc., 1988, 345.

7. Ibid., 5.

8. "A Multicenter Evaluation of a Proprietary Weight Reduction Program for the Treatment of Marked Obesity." The Journal of The American Medical Association 268 (1992): 3307.

9. Wysong, R. L. "Natural vs. Technological Foods." *Wysong Review.* Midland, MI: Wysong Institute, January, 1988.

10. Benum, Sara. "Feast or Famine." Complementary Medicine 2.3 (January-February, 1987): 14.

11. Bouchard, Claude. "Is Weight Fluctuation a Risk Factor?" The New England Journal of Medicine 324 (1991): 1887.

12. MacEwen, Gregory, VMD. "Fat Cats and Dogs." Petfood Industry 31.4 (July-August, 1989): 28.

13. Ibid.

14. Kronfeld, D.S., DVM, Ph.D. "Veterinary Supervised Weight Reduction Program Can Scale Down Pounds For Overweight Canines." DVM, The Newsmagazine of Veterinary Medicine 19.7 (July 1988): 60.

3 - THE MIRACLE OF WEIGHT MAINTENANCE

The maintenance of normal weight depends upon a myriad of complex and inter-related factors

All species of life, plant and animal, have their own "normal" average weight-to-height ratio. This provides a range of normalcy. Below this range, life can be threatened due to insufficient weight. Above it, life can be jeopardized by excessive weight.

On the surface, it seems to be a simple matter. If weight is insufficient, simply consume more and/or expend less. If weight is excessive, simply consume less and/or expend more. But maintaining a normal range of weight depends upon an incredibly complex labyrinth of physiology and biochemistry that, once distorted, is not easily resolved for a growing segment of human and companion-animal populations.

Normal weight is more incredible than abnormal weight

Remaining within a normal weight range is natural and automatic — given our natural synorgonic context. In this context, no decision has to be made as to how much or how little to eat, or how active or inactive to be. Genetically programmed systems are in place to turn appetite on and off, to increase desire for certain types of food and reject others, to absorb nutrients as needed and to excrete those which are not needed, and to adjust metabolism and energy expenditures to meet demands that range from sleeping to running a marathon.

Body levels of nitrogen, minerals and electrolytes are amazingly stable with daily uptake usually equal to excretion. When we eat what hunger dictates and expend energy as we desire, a balance is maintained. It is not unusual for a 160-pound adult human to maintain normal weight, give or take five pounds, throughout a lifetime.

Considering the wide range of variables which can affect an organism through the

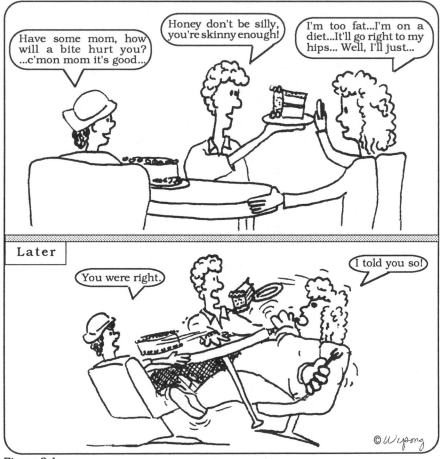

Figure 3-1

course of its life, it is indeed a wonder that weight can often be maintained within narrow ranges. If it were up to volition alone, inevitable errors about what and when to eat, and about how much energy to expend, would create populations made up of extremes — skin and bones on the one hand, and flabby balloons on the other. A few peanuts a day for example, in addition to normal meals, would create several additional pounds in a few years. Life itself would be threatened without precise innate controls.

If permitted, children can self-regulate food consumption

Children demonstrate these natural controls remarkably well. What appears to be an erratic and capricious appetite has been shown in controlled scientific studies to carefully regulate food intake to energy needs regardless of activity. After studying the remarkable correlation between food intake and metabolic requirements in children given free choice in food selection, one researcher remarked, "It would seem that natural habits have been operating efficiently for many millennia in ways not completely understood by nutritionists who are of more recent origin."

All that coaxing, bribing, cajoling and threatening does little to assure good nutrition for our children who are still tuned in, not yet having their synorgonic senses dulled. In contrast, we modern adults no longer listen to the inner voices but rather use modern food abundance as a recreational passport to obesity.

As the various factors which interrelate to maintain weight within normal limits are

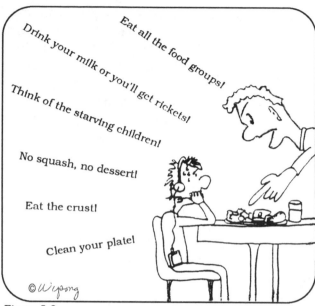

Eat all the food groups!

Drink your milk or you'll get rickets!

Think of the starving children!

No squash, no dessert!

Eat the crust!

Clean your plate!

© Wypong

Figure 3-2

Weight main-tenance touches virtually all the body's metabolic functions

considered in the following chapters, it will become apparent that with such complexity there is ample room for error, breakdown, mishap, and imbalance. Normalcy will seem more remarkable than aberration. The poor success rate in treating the puzzling disorder of obesity becomes understandable.

Weight maintenance touches virtually every metabolic system within the body in one way or another. It is thus dependent upon the proper integrated functioning of literally millions of complex biochemical interactions. Obesity is not therefore a unitary disorder. It calls into play the brain and neurotransmitters, the gut and peptides, the liver and its metabolic processes, adipose tissue and hormones. With such complexities, and the human proclivity to interfere with natural cycles, it is little wonder indeed that weight problems exist and that simplistic quick fixes do not resolve the problem.

The problem of obesity is deep seated and philosophically rooted in where we stand in the stream of time.

———————————

4 - OUR GENETIC ROOTS

Obesity follows the development of industrialized society

Obesity occurs primarily as a result of humans intervening in natural synorgonic cycles. We and the animals under our care have been extracted from our environmental roots, placed in new artificial settings, and subjected to new synthetic conditions. Refrigerators and cupboards full, cheap fast food, convenient junk food, abundant leisure, and easily accessible transportation and shelter are products of a rotund society — and so is abundant fat.

The disparity between what we need for survival and what we take is outrageous. We need about 2,300 calories per day in food to sustain ourselves, but on the average use 230,000 calories in food, fuel products, etc. to maintain our modern synthetic lifestyles.[1]

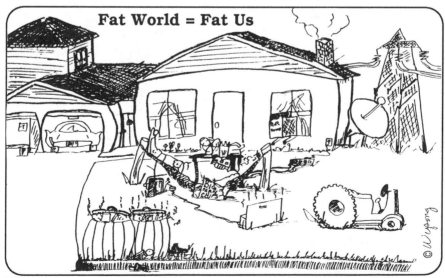

Figure 4-1

In the wild, given life outdoors and the only food being that which is found in nature, obesity is practically nonexistent. Birds, ants, salmon, racoons, tigers, elephants and seals all have a remarkable uniformity within their species. Compare this with the incredible variety in size among humans found on any public beach, and the key to the problem becomes apparent. Starvation can, of course, occur in the wild, but it is simply a function

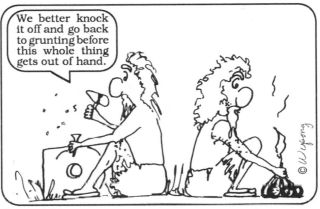

Figure 4-2

The
modern
setting
has
removed
us from
our
genetic
design

of insufficient food sources. It is not an eating disorder such as anorexia (self-forced starvation) or bulimia (forced vomiting). Neither humans nor animals in the wild experience the weight problems characteristic of modern society. The problem is obviously linked to modern society.[2,3]

It is easy to lose sight of the distance created between us and our natural context. In the wild we would be outdoors most of the time. In a pre-industrial setting we would also breathe clean, fresh air, drink pure, non-polluted water, and eat fresh, whole, raw foods as they came from the vine, so to speak.   In this natural setting, we would need to expend considerable effort in order to obtain little.   Exercise and a moderate food supply would prevail, unlike leisure and food abundance, which are the order of today's world.

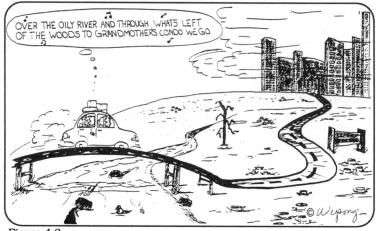

Figure 4-3

Modern life subjects us to a new, synthetic environment

In the modern world we live in, our homes are fabricated of synthetic materials gassing off various chemicals. We live under artificial fluorescent and incandescent spectrum modified light. We breathe industrially polluted air, travel by automatic vehicles rather than under our own power, go long stretches of time without any lengthy exposure to the sun, and drink water tainted by synthetic additives and pollutants.   We eat foods that are embalmed and artifact-based which bear little resemblance to anything that could be called "natural food," and we subject ourselves to a wide range of urban stresses with little opportunity to react (the fight-or-flight reaction, for example) to these stresses as we are naturally designed to do.

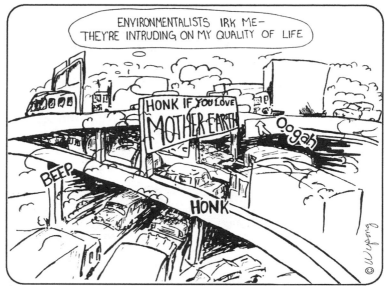

Figure 4-4

These dramatic alterations have occurred within an amazingly brief period of time. To put this in vivid perspective, one could draw a timeline 276 miles long, illustrating by scale a common estimate for the duration of life on Earth. On this scale, only one inch out of the entire 276 miles would represent the brief time span during which humans and animals have been eating modern, processed so-called scientifically designed foods.

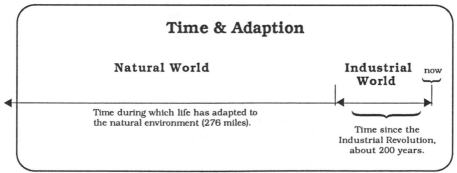

Figure 4-5

The introduction of modern, processed foods, their abundance, and the thousands of chemical additives used and created in their production, is a gigantic experiment in which we have all been the unwitting subjects. The complete results of this experiment are unknown. Many results that are known are not encouraging (see Figure 4-7).

We are all part of a gigantic experiment

When a child is born, it comes into the world fully expecting the environment of the 276 miles, to literally drop out on the forest floor, so to speak. Instead, it is subjected to something entirely different: the environment of the latest inch.

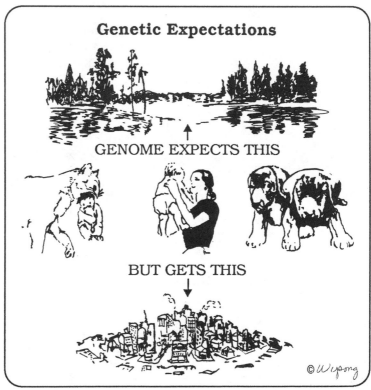

Figure 4-6

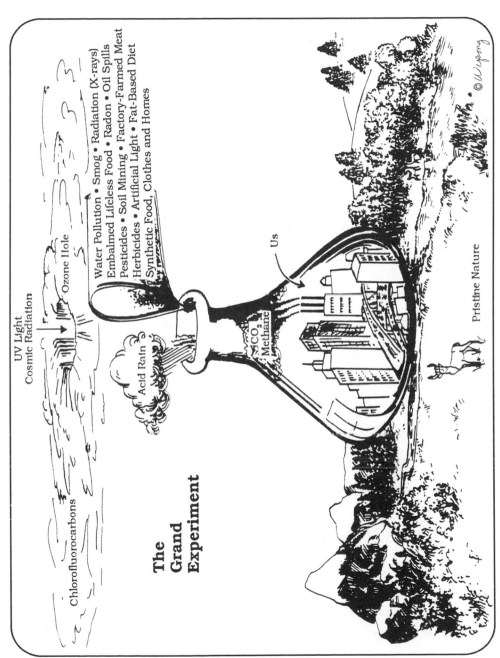

UV Light
Cosmic Radiation

Chlorofluorocarbons

Ozone Hole

Acid Rain

Water Pollution • Smog • Radiation (X-rays)
Embalmed Lifeless Food • Radon • Oil Spills
Pesticides • Soil Mining • Factory-Farmed Meat
Herbicides • Artificial Light • Fat-Based Diet
Synthetic Food, Clothes and Homes

CO_2
Methane

Us

The
Grand
Experiment

Pristine Nature

Figure 4-7

We develop and transmit an external material culture independent of internal genetic considerations. We thus find ourselves in a genetic time warp. We're in one place; our genes are in another. Our genes are adapted to a natural, pristine environment, a life of exercise, and natural, whole, raw foods, but we find ourselves somewhere else.

We are in a genetic time warp

We are increasingly making ourselves like fish out of water. We drain our own pond, saw through the limb we sit on, and foul our own nest.

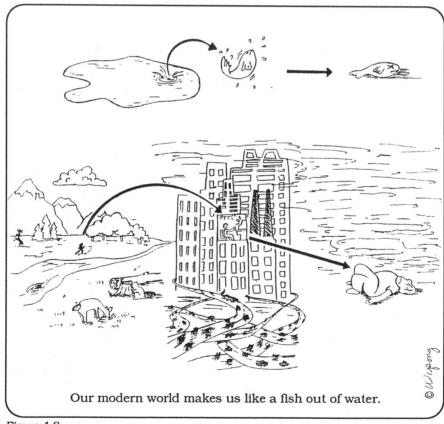

Our modern world makes us like a fish out of water.

Figure 4-8

Obesity is, in part, a failure to adapt properly to our new, synthetic world

We are making ourselves like E. T. aliens on our own planet. It's kind of like foolishly removing our spacesuits if we visited another planet. But it's different. Stupider. We're changing our planet such that we'll all need spacesuits to survive here. We are disengaging ourselves from our own life support systems.

The wide range of alterations we have made in our environment does not go without notice by our organism, which is designed, in effect, for a different world. The net difference

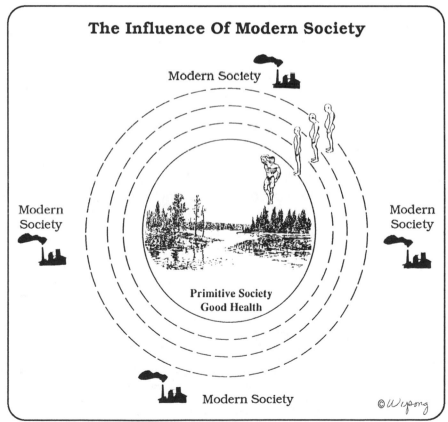

Figure 4-9

between being in full accord with our environment, and the degree of failure to adapt to it equals susceptibility to disease — such as obesity.

Under-standing our place within synorgon is the key to health

But the imperative is to survive, so our bodies attempt to adapt. However, we are capable of doing only so much. Each organism has its own biochemical weaknesses and capabilities. Some are very adaptable, and others are susceptible even to minor alterations from the natural balances. The effects are broad and complex. They constitute either overt or incubating disease (dis-ease with our environment). In fact, it is now estimated that more than 80 percent of all modern deaths occur as a result of our inability to adapt to the new world we have created.[4] This estimate is probably conservative.

Seeing our appropriate place within synorgon (which is really not so much a place as an unobtrusive presence in an intricate dynamic web) provides the necessary clue to understanding why many diseases, including obesity, occur, and what can be done to prevent or reverse them.

---

1. Hardin, Garrett, "There is no global population problem." An audio tape produced by The American Humanist Association, Amherst, N.Y.
2. Frankle, Reva T., and Yang, Mei-Uih. *Obesity and Weight Control: The Health Professional's Guide to Understanding and Treatment.* Gaithersburg: Aspen Publishers, 1988.
3. Eaton, S. Boyd, M.D., and Konner, Melvin, Ph.D. "Paleolithic Nutrition: A Consideration of Its Nature and Current Implications." The New England Journal of Medicine 312 (1985): 283-289.
4. "Prevention of Cancer." Science 182 (1973): 4116.

Though normally viewed as a personal, cosmetic or health problem, both the causes and the results of obesity reach much further. One of the best ways to understand how obesity is an interconnected issue is to see its environmental implications.

We live in a world of finite resources and swelling populations. Given this, it does not seem appropriate that 60 million people a year die of starvation, while almost 100 million adults and young people, in the United States alone, consume far in excess of their needs.

Obesity takes a toll both on individual health and on the environment

This is not to suggest that if we ate less, people would no longer starve elsewhere in the world. It might help — not only others but us — but world hunger is a far more complex issue. Problems of distribution, greed and political stalemate often thwart feeding the hungry. But, the fact of the matter is that there is plenty of cropland to feed the Earth's population many times over. If so, where is all the excess food going while millions starve?

Some of it is going on our bodies. Much of it, however, is being inefficiently and unnecessarily converted into animal-based foods.

Excess fat on people comes primarily from the excess consumption not of plant products, but of meat products. It is difficult (if not impossible) to find an obese person whose diet is solely vegetation based. Our rolls,

29

dimples and bulges were literally once the rolls, dimples and bulges of poultry, cattle, and pigs. As we will discuss in a later chapter, the fat of animals quite efficiently and directly becomes ours.

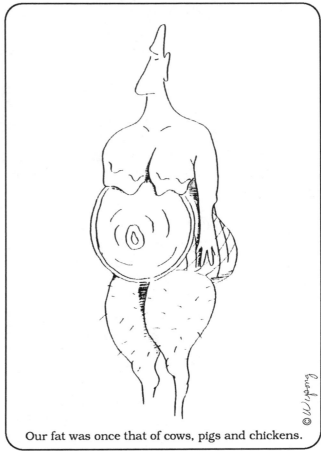

Our fat was once that of cows, pigs and chickens.

Figure 5-1

Not only is excess meat consumption a ticket to obesity and a robber of health, but the world's glut of flesh squanders resources significantly and pollutes, jeopardizing the health of all life on Earth.

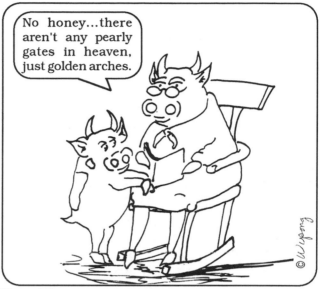

Figure 5-2

The production of animal meats squanders resources

For cxample, twenty pounds of grain can either directly feed humans, or be inefficiently used to create one pound of beef. In order to make the meat conversion, vast

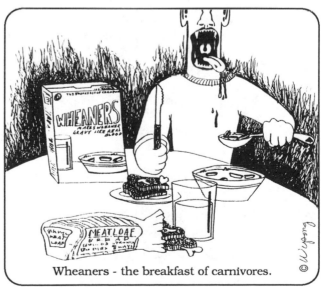

Figure 5-3

amounts of farmland are used to grow the excess grains necessary to create flesh. It takes 75 times more land to feed the same number of people beef as opposed to rice. Put another way, the resources used to feed 210 million Americans a meat-based diet could feed 1.5 billion Chinese their vegetation-based diet.

The energy to produce one hamburger could feed 100 third-world people

Hidden in this inefficiency is also the environmental toll of the millions of tons of fertilizer and pesticides used to grow crops, as well as the fossil fuels necessary to work the land, transport, cool, and freeze the meats. The energy used to produce, package, cool, and transport one hamburger could create food to feed 100 third-world people. The waste due to the inefficiency of converting vegetable products to meat products is so profound that if the consumption of animal products was curtailed for just one day a week in the U.S. alone, the 60 million people

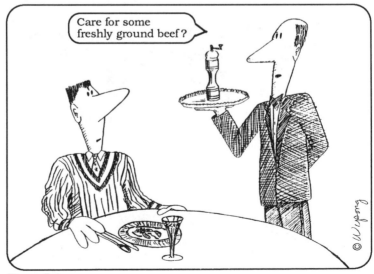

Figure 5-4

who starve each year world-wide could be fed (provided the food value could be properly distributed to them, of course).

An emphasis on meat products degrades the environment and encourages obesity

Ruminants, such as cows and sheep, also create methane, a greenhouse gas, and produce waste which, instead of being used to fertilize producing land, ends up polluting ground water and tributaries. Consider also that our oxygen-producing rainforests (the Earth's lungs) are being razed in part to create pasture for hamburger-producing cattle. The land required here is not negligible. In fact, it takes approximately 55 square feet of rainforest to make one hamburger. In addition, more than 5,000 gallons of water (an amount greater than that which each of us uses in a year to shower) are required to produce one pound of meat. One half of the entire U.S. water supply is used in animal product production.[1,2] Such are the sweeping consequences of a palate conditioned to meat and fat.

Excess fat contributes to the world's energy deficit

It is estimated that there are as many as three billion excess pounds of fat deposited on the American population. This excess fat represents in energy approximately six trillion kilocalories. This is the potential energy in one and a half billion gallons of gasoline — sufficient energy to power about a million automobiles per year, or provide the total annual electrical needs of Boston, Chicago, San Francisco, and Washington, D.C.[3]

Added to these considerations are the peripheral costs of putting on these extra pounds. There is the energy required to produce, transport, refrigerate and package the animal food products; travel cost for people to purchase them; disposal of the waste; outfitting of reducing centers; transportation of people to these centers; and all the medical costs for resultant problems. The true price for society, the world, and the environment is staggering.

Considering its environmental toll, obesity is not a private matter

Obesity is not really a private matter.

Additionally, when we begin to see ourselves as simply a part of our world and not as a specially commissioned apex predator, the factory farming of animals raises ethical questions. Deforesting, strip mining and polluting are manifestations of the same insensitivity required for confining veal calves, caging chickens and pigs and shooting animals for

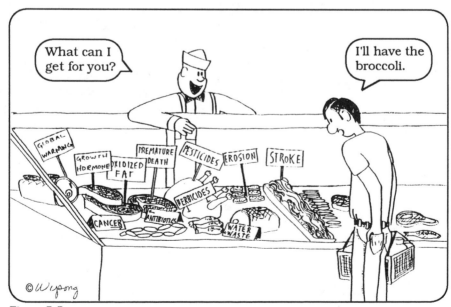

Figure 5-5

"sport." Killing one another is murder while doing it to other creatures for money or fun is condoned.

This is not to say that all meat eating is wrong. Evidence in support of meat eating can also be argued. Every primitive society ever studied ate meat, and primitive societies do not suffer from obesity or other degenerative diseases. Eating food based upon what our food "feels" does not create clear choices. There are no distinct lines between life forms to demarcate that which is sentient and does not feel pain and that which does.

Additionally, some people may not fare well nutritionally with a total vegetation-based diet depending upon whether they are descendents of a vegetarian-based or meat-based society. For example, Asians (vegetarian heritage) may not be able to tolerate milk, whereas many Africans and Europeans (herd heritage) thrive on it. (See *The Wysong Review*, July 1992, for a more thorough discussion of carnivorism vs. vegetarianism - page 258.

I know this is an emotionally charged issue. Hunters may love their sport, farmers love their occupation and vegans (vegetables only — no meat, dairy or eggs) love their compassion for animals. Nutritionists may say there are elements in meat (vitamin B_{12}, certain amino acids, etc.) necessary for our health, anatomists argue about whether the length of our intestinal tract is vegetarian or carnivorous, and health researchers cite the

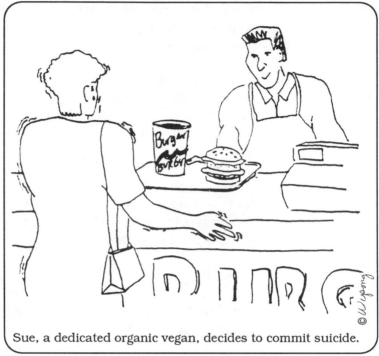

Sue, a dedicated organic vegan, decides to commit suicide.

Figure 5-6

decreased incidence of certain diseases in vegetarians.

It's confusing to say the least. Although everyone seems to have a strong view on what should or should not be eaten, few form these beliefs for the right reason. Emotion, bias, irrationality, greed, fear and love dictate choices rather than reason and foresight. Long-range health, both for ourselves and the Earth, should be the guiding principle.

It is certain that the amount of meat western societies consume is excessive and that more sensitivity toward other species and the planet at large is necessary if we are to live in healthy synorgonic balance and leave a sustainable planet to our children. (More specific guidelines on how to achieve this balance through food choices will be discussed in Section II.)

Understanding the limits of our finite world, the need not to squander resources and the responsibility to protect our environment are sufficient reasons in themselves to make every effort to maintain appropriate weight by not only reducing consumption, but also by shifting more to vegetation-based foods.

---

1. Lefferts, Lisa Y. and Blobaum, Roger. "Eating as if the Earth Mattered." The Environmental Magazine, Vol. III, No. 1 (Jan./Feb. 1992): 31-37.
2. Robbins, John. "Can Earth Survive the Big Mac Attack?" The Environmental Magazine, Vol. III, No. 1 (Jan./Feb. 1992): 38-43, 60-61.
3. Hannon, B.M. and Lohman, T.G. "The Energy Cost of Overweight in the United States." American Journal of Public Health 68: 765.

If the environmental issues are not sufficient reason, the direct health consequences of obesity should be enough to give anyone pause to reflect.

Obesity adversely affects virtually every organ system. The following is a sobering list of disease conditions directly related to excess weight. These pathologies are common to both obese humans and animals. They make it clear that the more weight that is carried, the less time there will be to carry it.

The more weight carried, the less time there is to carry it

1. Hypertension (high blood pressure due to vascular disease and high blood sodium)
2. Adult-onset diabetes (a result of increased insulin resistance − the body adapts to excess food by making tissues more resistant to uptake of excess nutrients such as glucose)
3. Various dermatoses (skin disorders)
4. Hypercholesterolemia (high blood cholesterol)
5. Hypertriglyceridemia (high blood triglycerides)
6. Atherosclerosis (associated with decreased HDL-cholesterol levels and leading to peripheral vascular disease, heart attacks and strokes)
7. Varicose veins
8. Clumsiness and decreased agility
9. Susceptibility to accidents
10. Arthritis and other bone and joint disorders
11. Sterility

12. Obstetrical problems
13. Hormonal abnormalities (increased estrogen levels in both men and women; dysfunctional uterine bleeding, amenorrhea, inadequate luteal phase, breast and endometrial cancer in women; low testosterone in men)
14. Gallstones
15. Gout
16. Delayed healing
17. Increased susceptibility to stress
18. Increased risk in surgery
19. Nutritional deficiencies (often the foods that are eaten in excess are nutrient poor)
20. Decreased glucose tolerance (associated with hypoglycemia and diabetes)
21. Decreased respiratory efficiency (blood CO_2 levels rise because of the inability to sufficiently lift the chest wall, which can in turn lead to increased lethargy and somnolence)
22. Polycythemia (an excess level of red blood cells) and thrombosis (blood clot formation)
23. Increased incidence of obesity in offspring
24. Increased incidence of cancer in offspring
25. Increased mortality rate of most conditions, sudden death, and decreased life-span
26. Increased sweating (due to decreased skin-to-body-mass ratio)
27. Snoring
28. Fat-fold dermatitis
29. Increased left ventricular mass (leading to stroke, congestive heart failure, hypertension, and cardiomyopathy)
30. Anorexia nervosa and/or bulimia
31. Psychosocial disorders[1-20]

Even the susceptibility to environmental toxins increases with obesity. For example, DDT, though banned in the U.S. in 1972, is present in every person's fat stores. DDT, like PCB, dioxin and other highly toxic chlorinated organics, is fat soluble. The more fat carried, the greater the levels of such fat soluble pollutants. Now, decades after the ban, it is found that DDT mimics estrogen in women and can promote breast cancer.[21]

Advanced age and obesity are not seen together

Obesity strains the adaptive capabilities of organisms. Just one pound of additional fat requires three additional miles of capillaries to supply it. The burden compounds with every pound gained, pushing health toward the disease precipice. Sufficiently strained by simply maintaining the increased mass, the body has little reserve left to combat infections and metabolic or emotional stress. Unhealthiness is the inevitable consequence. Decreasing fat intake to 30 percent of calories could save some 42,000 lives a year. However, a greater reduction in fat intake would be ideal.[22]

The physical consequences of obesity are often obvious and usually are the focus of complaints and therapy. In our mechanistic, repair-oriented society, it is easy to forget that such physical problems are attached to real, feeling people. To the majority of health professionals and the public, obesity is simply seen as a need for the patient to muster the will to control his or her own gluttony. Obese people — in the mind of the unenlightened critic — are therefore failures and deserving of social contempt.[23]   The social, psychological, and emotional tolls may be the worst tragedies of all for the obese. As one surgeon writes:

The emotional conse- quences of obesity may exact the biggest price of all

"The emotional cost of morbid obesity is also enormous. Obese patients are often unable to fit into armchairs, find suitable clothing, obtain access to public toilets, and enter public convey- ances. If they can enter an automo- bile, they may be unable to get out. Employers usually consider the mor- bidly obese poor risks because of unfa- vorable appearance, inability to fit into office furniture or into factory environ- ments, and high absenteeism due to illness. In relationships with their peers, the severely obese make few friendships and seldom find satisfac- tory marital or sexual partners, al- though the libidos of these obese indi- viduals are often as great as their size. Obese women, particularly, tend to marry inadequate spouses who are afraid to accept the challenge of more desirable females. The object of jokes, the morbidly obese play the role of the jolly fat person, hiding their misery in public and soothing it by eating even more. In short, they are generally very unhappy people indeed, emotionally deprived and physically handi- capped."[24]

With such terrible consequences, obesity should be addressed before it ever begins.

When obesity is present, every effort should be made to reverse it. It is not simply a matter of cosmetics or individual lifestyle choice. It is a serious disease condition that wreaks pain, incapacity and death.

Not everyone who is overweight is doomed, however. Although in the minority, some do escape complications from obesity for some unknown reason. It is also true that for some causes of mortality, the lean are more at risk than the obese. Though this may be true, it should not be taken to repudiate obesity's dangers any more than a 90-year-old smoker should calm our fears about smoking. It can also be noted that some people drive drunk repeatedly for a lifetime without consequence, and some on the front line of a military action survive. This does not make such choices wise.

Disease in the lean does not deny the greater dangers for the obese

We do not have to understand all the consequences of increased weight to desire to be in a normal weight range. People are well aware of obesity, and they expend considerable effort attempting to reverse it for themselves, their children, and their companion animals. Most people understand that obesity limits life, is aesthetically unpleasant, and predisposes them to various diseases. Nobody chooses to be obese.

Unfortunately, efforts to reverse obesity are often as philosophically distorted as the causes. Obesity is, by and large, a departure from natural lifestyles and food sources. Its cause is, in part, the pleasure of ease. With

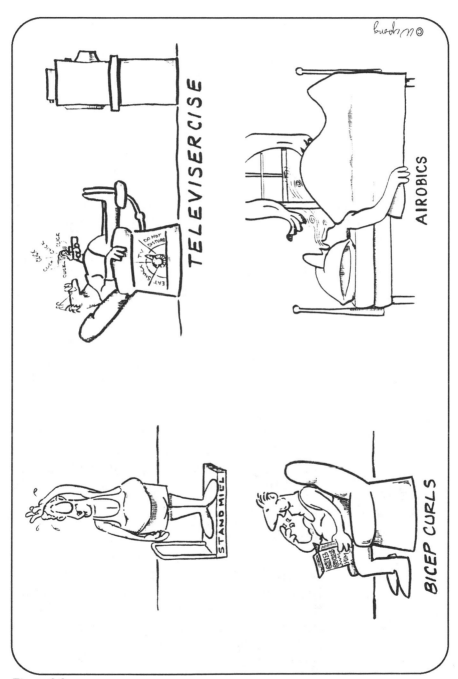

Figure 6-1

Ease lies at the root of some weight problems and is used in vain to solve them

Taking personal charge, not relying on experts or products, is key to solving weight problems

that in mind, many programs designed to help the obese are designed with ease as the number one feature. There are exercise salons with machines to move body parts for you, diet pills to suppress hunger, reducing candy bars and milkshakes, and fad programs emphasizing single foods such as grapefruit or popcorn. Changing is difficult and requires effort, whereas buying a pill, a membership or an ice-cream-flavored drink is easy, and fits within the same old comfortable life patterns.

Furthermore, obesity is something more than that which can be repaired by someone else with a silver bullet or bandage. Our society has become used to relying on experts and professionals to solve our every need. Arguments are solved in court, wages are negotiated by unions, teeth are cleaned by dentists, foods are grown and prepared by others, blocked arteries are roto-rooted by surgeons, and a damaged heart is simply replaced. We have come to believe that all problems we experience can be solved by technology and experts in our modern society. They cannot.

It is unfortunate that the consequences of obesity are delayed until the obesity has become deeply ingrained. If a significant painful consequence resulted the moment the body became overweight, an appropriate pain reflex would result, prompting discontinuance of whatever patterns were leading to the obesity. We learn quickly not to put our hand into an open flame, for example. But,

Delay in the obesity pain reflex fools us

as with many other chronic, degenerative diseases, the cause is often far removed from the result. Thus, it is easy to be fooled that the two are unrelated. This is the insidious danger in seemingly innocuous recreational activities such as overeating, smoking, and drinking.

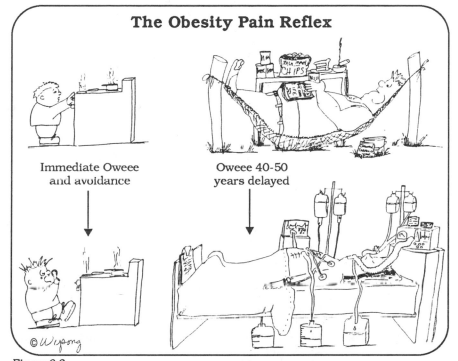

The Obesity Pain Reflex

Immediate Oweee and avoidance

Oweee 40-50 years delayed

© Wysong

Figure 6-2

The same intelligence which can ruin must be used to save

A new approach to living is in order. It is one based on individual action, on respect for natural balances, on fiduciary responsibility, and on self improvement with prevention as the primary goal.

The mind can indeed be a ruinous tenant of its landlord, the body. But the same mind, the intelligence and will which has created a society of toxins and excesses, now must be used to recognize long-term harm, and make the salutary adjustments.

———————

1. DeFronzo, R. A., et al. Journal of Clinical Investigation 58 (1976): 83-89.
2. Maclure, K. Malcom, Sc.D., et al. "Weight, Diet, and the Risk of Symptomatic Gallstones in Middle-Aged Women." The New England Journal of Medicine 321 (1989): 563.
3. Council on Scientific Affairs. "Treatment of Obesity in Adults." The Journal of the American Medical Association 260 (1988): 2547-2551.
4. DeFronzo, R. A., et al. Journal of Clinical Investigation 58 (1976): 83-89.
5. Pi-Sunyer, F. Xavier. *Modern Nutrition in Health and Disease.* Philadelphia: Lea & Febiger, 1988, p. 802.
6. Raloff, J. "Mom's Fatty Diet May Induce Child's Cancer." Science News 137 (1990): 5.
7. Peterson, Hugh R., M.D., et al. "Body Fat and the Activity of the Autonomic Nervous System." The New England Journal of Medicine 318 (1988): 1077.
8. Armstrong, D.B., et al. The Journal of the American Medical Association 147 (1951): 1007-1014.
9. Lew, E. A. Journal of the American Dietetic Association 38 (1961): 323-327.
10. Build and Blood Pressure Study, 1959. Vol 1. Chicago: Society of Actuaries, 1960.
11. Build Study, 1979. Chicago: Society of Actuaries and Association of Life Insurance Medical Directors, 1980.
12. Schneider, G., et al. "Increased estrogen production in obese men." Journal of Clinical Endocrinol Metabolism 48 (1979): 633.
13. The American Journal of Clinical Nutrition. Supplement to 53-6.
14. Sorlie, P., et al. "Body build and mortality: the Framingham Study." The Journal of the American Medical Association 243 (1980): 1828-1831.
15. Tobian, L. "Hypertension and obesity." The New England Journal of Medicine 298 (1978): 46-48.
16. Kannel, W.B., et al. "The relation of adiposity to blood pressure and development of hypertension: the Framingham Study." Ann Intern Med. 67 (1967): 48-59.
17. Ostlund, R.E., Jr., et al. "The ratio of waist-to-hip circumference, plasma insulin level, and glucose intolerance as independent predictor of the HDL cholesterol level in older adults." The New England Journal of Medicine 322 (1990): 229-234.

18. Alexander, J.K. "The cardiomyopathy of obesity." Pro-gressive Cardiovascular Disease 27 (1985): 325-334.
19. Colditz, Graham A., et al. "Diet and risk of clinical diabetes in women." The American Journal of Clinical Nutrition 55 (1992): 1018.
20. Schapira, David V., MBChB, et al. "Upper-Body Fat Distribution and Endometrial Cancer Risk." The Journal of the American Medical Association 266 (1991): 1808.
21. Raloff, J. "DDT may foster breast cancer, study finds." Science News 143 (1993): 262.
22. Browner, Warren S., M.D., et al. "What If Americans Ate Less Fat?" The Journal of the American Medical Association 265 (1991): 3288.
23. Frankle, Reva T. and Yang, Mei-Uih. *Obesity and Weight Control.* Maryland: Aspen Publishers, 1988.
24. Pories, Walter J., M.D. "The Surgical Approach to Morbid Obesity" in *Textbook of Surgery - The Biological Basis of Modern Surgical Practice.* Philadelphia: W. B. Saunders, 1991, pp. 851-866.

7 - MEASURING FAT

Determining obesity is difficult if left to the individual in question. We play cat-and-mouse games of deception. Being "pleasantly plump" or having a "large frame" or being "big boned" are comfortable euphemisms for obesity. We tend to seek out friends who are like us and who minimize any problems we may have. We buy scales that underweigh, try putting the scale on a deep pile carpet to knock some pounds off, pull in our stomachs, tighten our belts, and find charts and literature that assuage our fears about reality. But most of us, if we permit ourselves to be objective, know if we are overweight or not.

Standard charts, such as the one on page 49, help determine normal weight based on an individual's height and age. There are also sophisticated methods of measuring fat percentages, including skin-fold calipers, hydrostatic procedures, electro-bioimpedance, and the measurement of fat-soluble gases, such as krypton, and xenon.[1-2] The height-to-weight charts and skinfold measurements (known as anthropometric measures) are the most usual forms of measuring body fat levels in humans.[3]

A rule of thumb to follow to determine normal weight is that for women, weight should be height in inches times 3.5 minus 108. For men it should be height times 4.0 minus 128. Depending upon the basic skeletal frame, normalcy can range from 4 percent under to 8 percent over these values.

Determine Your Ideal Weight Range
Measure your wrist to determine your frame size

WOMEN	
Small	5 to 5-1/2 inch wrist
Medium	5-1/2 to 6 inch wrist
Large	6 to 6-1/2 inch wrist

MEN	
Small	6-1/2 to 7 inch wrist
Medium	7 to 7-1/2 inch wrist
Large	7-1/2 to 8 inch wrist

Height and Weight Table

MEN

Height Feet	Inches	Small Frame	Medium Frame	Large Frame
5	2	128-134	131-141	138-150
5	3	130-136	133-143	140-153
5	4	132-138	135-145	142-156
5	5	134-140	137-148	144-160
5	6	136-142	139-151	146-164
5	7	138-145	142-154	149-168
5	8	140-148	145-157	152-172
5	9	142-151	148-160	155-176
5	10	144-154	151-163	158-180
5	11	146-157	154-166	161-184
6	0	149-160	157-170	164-188
6	1	152-164	160-174	168-192
6	2	155-168	164-178	172-197
6	3	158-172	167-182	176-202
6	4	162-176	171-187	181-207

WOMEN

Height Feet	Inches	Small Frame	Medium Frame	Large Frame
4	10	102-111	109-121	118-131
4	11	103-113	111-123	120-134
5	0	104-115	113-126	122-137
5	1	106-118	115-129	125-140
5	2	108-121	118-132	128-143
5	3	111-124	121-135	131-147
5	4	114-127	124-138	134-151
5	5	117-130	127-141	137-155
5	6	120-133	130-144	140-159
5	7	123-136	133-147	143-163
5	8	126-139	136-150	146-167
5	9	129-142	139-153	149-170
5	10	132-145	142-156	152-173
5	11	135-148	145-159	155-176
6	0	138-151	148-162	158-179

Height indicates subjects are wearing shoes with 1-inch heels or less. Weights reflect adults age 25 to 59 years and are based on lowest mortality.

Figure 7-1

In general, people who are honest with themselves can strip in front of a mirror and easily recognize whether they are carrying extra weight or not.

A mirror is an excellent analytical tool for obesity

As little as 10 percent over ideal weight is considered by most medical experts to constitute obesity. Objectively take the measure, and if you are overweight, face the reality and the seriousness of the disease you have. This honesty is an essential first step in the Synorgon Diet. If you are obese, it is not time to despair, get depressed, and go raid the cupboard because you're doomed. Identifying a problem is one of the most important solutions.

As you read further and deepen your understanding of your condition, you will see that there is hope. You can lose the weight, keep it off for a lifetime, and enjoy the exhilaration of having won a difficult battle. You can also look forward to a life of renewed health, energy, and vitality.

---

1. Benum, Sara. "Feast or Famine." Complementary Medicine, Healthcomm, Inc. 2 (Jan-Feb., 1987): 11.
2. Council on Scientific Affairs, "Treatment of Obesity in Adults." The Journal of the American Medical Association 260 (1988): 2547-2551.
3. Pi-Sunyer, F. Xavier. *Modern Nutrition In Health And Disease*, Philadelphia: Lea & Febiger, Philadelphia, 1988, p. 797.

8 - LIPIDS

To broaden your understanding of obesity, let's look more closely at just exactly what fat is. Just like getting to know a supposed enemy more closely often makes him a friend, so too will a more accurate knowledge of lipids (fats and oils) show them to be something far different from the demons we have come to fear and hate.

Lipids are not simply calories

Until relatively recently, lipids had been viewed as either providers of a protective and insulating layer for the body or as energy sources. However, as the modern diet has become further and further removed from its natural context through the use of processing, food fractions, and synthetic substitutions, various nutritional maladies aside from obesity have become linked to the consumption of lipids. Advances in research and analytical capabilities have made it possible to identify specific lipid factors in food which can affect health in profound and far-reaching ways.

Certain lipids are essential to health

Far from being just an inert food component, calorie source or organ pad, lipids have emerged as extremely complex dynamic biochemicals linked directly or indirectly to virtually every structure and metabolic function in the body. Lipids comprise a major component of the intricate structure of cell and organelle (organs within the cell) membranes. Therefore, they control the integrity of tissues and affect the flux of life-giving chemicals in and out of the cell. In addition, they serve as precursors for various hormones as well as highly reactive eicosanoids (autocoids) — hormone-like substances that regulate moment-by-moment function at the cellular level.

Considerable reseach has focused on fats in the diet, especially after it was determined that high serum cholesterol levels in humans were associated with cardiovascular disease. Recommendations were then made to decrease the intake of fats and cholesterol. This concept was embraced as a marketing opportunity by commercial interests who have now for many years argued the merits of "low cholesterol," "low fat," and "highly polyunsaturated" products.

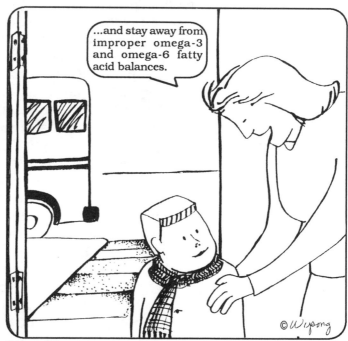

Figure 8-1

Recently, however, studies of certain cultures with high levels of fats in their diets without a concomitant high incidence of cardiovascular disease, and conflicting results of studies of populations in the U.S. itself, have created doubt that high fat and cholesterol necessarily cause cardiovascular disease. Current research has indicated that some societies with a low incidence of degenerative diseases were consuming not only high levels of fats (70 percent of calories — compared to the 30 percent consumed by Americans, which is considered excessive), but also relatively high levels of specific kinds of fats of the omega -3 and omega -9 families. These findings, combined with the discovery of the many biochemical actions of various fat metabolites, have created an exciting and promising new field in nutrition and health.[1-6]

Increased fat consumption does not necessarily mean disease

This is a new view of fat — one which promises health benefits, not simply lumps and bulges to burn off on a treadmill.

A confusing dilemma results. On the one hand, fat is anathema, something to rid from our diets and bodies; on the other, it is essential to life itself and may prevent certain diseases and improve the quality of health.

Lipid nutrition is a promising new field in health care

A basic understanding of the chemical nature of lipids is useful in appreciating their diverse role in metabolism and solving this apparent conundrum. For further details, refer to the three appendixes: "Lipid Biochemistry," "Lipid Digestion," and "Adipose Tissue," and my book *Lipid Nutrition: Understanding Fats and Oils in Health and Disease.*

Functions of Fatty Acids

FATTY ACID (FA)	FUNCTION/EFFECT
Medium-chain	Rapid energy; indicated in certain digestive malfunctions
Saturated	
Lauric (12:0)	Hyperlipidemic; hypercholesterolemic; prothrombotic
Myristic (14:0)	Dietary calories
Palmitic (16:0)	Dietary calories
Stearic (18:0)	Possibly hypolipidemic; precursor of oleic acid
Monounsaturated	
Oleic (18:1ω9)	Hypolipidemic/hypocholesterolemic; precursor of eicosatrienoic acid (20:3ω9) in essential fatty acid insufficiency
Erucic (22:1ω9)	Impaired fatty acid oxidation in heart of rat; common in rapeseed
ω6 polyunsaturated	
Linoleic (18:2ω6)	Component of acylglucosylceramides Precursor of arachidonic acid Hypolipidemic compared to saturated FA Increases membrane fluidity compared to saturated FA
γ-Linolenic (18:3ω6)	Precursor of eicosatrienoic acid and AA
γ-Homolinolenic (20:ω6)	Precursor of PGE1 series of eicosanoids
Arachidonic (AA;20:4ω6)	Membrane fluidity Precursor of eicosanoids
ω3 polyunsaturated	
α-Linolenic (18:3ω3)	Hypolipidemic Membrane fluidity Precursor of EPA and DHA (slow) Reduces eicosanoid synthesis
Eicosapentaenoic (EPA;20:5ω3)	Hypolipidemic Reduces AA synthesis and inflammatory eicosanoids Precursor of modulating eicosanoids
Docosahexaenoic (DHA;22:6ω3)	Hypolipidemic Important in vision and neural membranes Reduces AA synthesis and inflammatory eicosanoids

Figure 8-2

All readers should at least skim through these references to appreciate the intricate complexity of the fats and oils we consume and those retained within our bodies. Lipids are an essential part of our diet, our structure and function. Natural food lipids should not be omitted; but man-made lipids and processed, altered lipids must be shunned. In terms of removing us from our natural genetic context, the increased consumption of processed lipids is the most dramatic dieting change since the beginning of this century.[7] Such products are not foods — they are toxins perverting healthy tissue structures and disrupting critical metabolic functions. They are foreign to our synorgonic context, while natural lipids are a key component of the Synorgon Diet.

Immediately apply, as much as possible, this simple principle — welcome the lipids within raw natural foods and shun those which are fabricated or processed — to jump start yourself on the road to a healthier weight and life. In fact, for most obesity, this action in itself is the solution.

————————

1. Bang, H.O. and Dyerberg, J. "Lipid Metabolism and Ischemic Heart Disease in Greenland Eskimos." Adv. Lipid Res. 3 (1980): 1-22.
2. Sinclair, H.M. "The Diet of Canadian Indians and Eskimos." Proc. Nutr. Soc. 12 (1953): 69-82.
3. Kagawa, Y., et al. "Eicosapolyenoic Acids of Serum Lipids of Japanese Islanders With Low Incidence of Cardiovascular Diseases." J. Nutr. Sci. Vitaminaol 28 (1982): 441-453.
4. Hirai, A., et al. "Eicosapentaenoic Acid and Platelet Function in Japanese." The Lancet 2 (1980): 1132-1133.

5. Kromhout, D., et al. "The Inverse Relation Between Fish Consumption and 20-year Mortality From Coronary Heart Disease." The New England Journal of Medicine 312 (1985): 1205-1209.
6. Skekelle, R.B., et al. "Fish consumption and mortality from coronary heart disease." The New England Journal of Medicine 313 (1985): 820.
7. Tremblay, Angelo, et al. "Nutritional determinants of the increase in energy intake associated with a high-fat diet." American Journal of Clinical Nutrition 53 (1991): 1134.

9 - A CALORIE IS NOT A CALORIE

Energy is the stuff of life. Without consuming and utilizing energy, life simply is not possible. In a wild setting, which our genetic program still expects us to be in, we would simply listen to our inner signals and seek foods which stimulate taste, pleasure, and satiety.

Our "sweet" tooth" and "fat tooth" are survival tools abused in the modern setting

This built-in mechanism, not coincidentally, directs us to foodstuffs which will supply our energy needs. It is the reason that we have both a "sweet tooth" and a "fat tooth." Foods that are sweet contain energy-giving carbohydrates for moment-by-moment, more immediate needs. Fatty foods create a desirable mouthfeel and provide a concentrated energy source reserve within our body fat depots.

Fats contain more than twice the energy value of either proteins or carbohydrates. This is because they are fully reduced (containing as much chemical bond energy as is possible) and anhydrous (containing no water). Fats are hydrocarbon chains holding within them the energy from the sun in the form of chemical bonds. Being anhydrous, they are also capable of being more densely stored than hydrated (water-containing) molecules, such as carbohydrates.

Fat is the limousine of the food energy world. It is handled differently than other foodstuffs in terms of its digestion and metabolism. The high efficiency of its assimilation and storage contributes further to its energy potential compared to other foods.

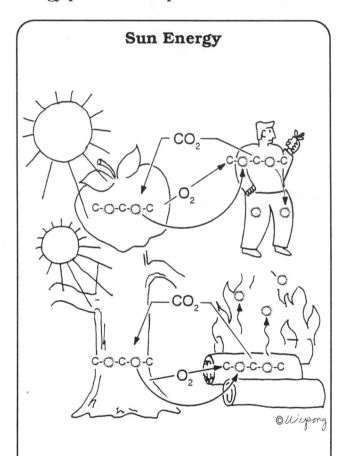

Sun Energy

Energy from the sun is converted and stored in carbon chains (C-O-C-O-C) in plants. These chains are found in carbohydrates and lipids. Once consumed, the chains are broken by use of oxygen, produced by plants, releasing the sun's energy for the body's needs. CO_2 is expired in the process. Similarly, wood is comprised of sun energy contained in carbon chains released as heat when wood is burned. Oxygen is consumed and CO_2 released in the process in the same way as in energy production in the body.

Figure 9-1

But conventional nutritional thinking commonly holds that a calorie is a calorie regardless of source. It is argued that if a food is burned in a laboratory bomb calorimeter (a device which measures the heat released by the combustion of a substance), and the number of calories is measured, the result quantitates all the energy that this food can deliver to the body.

Energy from a bomb calorimeter does not equate to the energy value utilized by the body

Such measurements find that fat contains about nine kilocalories per gram, whereas carbohydrate and protein each have about four kilocalories per gram. (One kilocalorie, also called calorie, is the energy necessary to raise the temperature of one gram of water one degree Celsius.) But think about it. What does raising the temperature of water one degree on a thermometer have to do with complex foods in complex bodies?

Herein lies the root of a nefarious problem in our approach to nutrition, medicine, and weight control. We reduce complex biological things to a mere assemblage of nuts, bolts, levers, pulleys, furnaces, and thermostats. It is naive and simplistic to believe complex foods in complex bodies behave like a food burnt in a furnace (bomb calorimeter).

We think this way because we understand machines. Of course we do; we make them. But we have not made living creatures, nor do we understand them.[1] We fool ourselves thinking that living creatures, humans, animals, and their foods are simple machines reducible to pieces and heat.

Why is this issue important? Because if nutritionists can get us to believe there are no differences between calories, then we will look at foods not as what they are, but as analytical values. This opens the door for endless food manipulation by processors. As long as the calories on a label meet a dietician's guidelines, then it doesn't really matter what the food is...or so they would have us believe.

In actual fact, it is the makeup, the very nature of and complexity within food, not its analytical value in calories, that determines our ability to maintain healthy weight.

Calories being equal, a high fat diet will result in the highest level of body fat deposition

The following discussion is meant to disprove the "calorie is a calorie regardless of source" myth and refocus attention on what food is in substance. This won't be popular with nutritionists who want you to believe they have everything all figured out, or with food processors who want to feed us high-profit fractionated refined embalmed pablum that is dyed, colored, and perfumed to make us believe it's real food.

In one study, for example, humans overfed a mixed diet took seven months to increase weight 30 pounds while another group overfed a high-fat diet took only three months to increase 30 pounds. Both groups received the same number of calories.[2] Also consider that Americans consume fewer calories, on the average, than the Chinese, but are typically much fatter.[3] This can be linked to the fact that American fat intake is much higher than that of the Chinese. In other studies it

The body can utilize 97 percent of fat calories but only 77 percent of carbohydrate calories

There is greater thermic loss with a carbohydrate meal than a lipid meal

has been found that obese individuals do not necessarily consume more calories than normal weight individuals.[4] In an animal study, one group of rats fed a high-fat diet ended up with 50 percent body fat, whereas those fed a high-carbohydrate diet ended up with 30 percent body fat.[5] Caloric intake was the same for both groups. Lipids indeed provide an energy storage edge beyond the number assigned to them from a laboratory bomb calorimeter.

Not all the energy from food consumed is available for use by the body. On the average, 65 percent of the energy from food that is digested and assimilated is used for resting metabolic functions; 15 percent is normally used for thermogenesis (the thermic energy required for digestion,[6,7] absorption, transport, and fueling the sodium/potassium pump in tissues); and approximately 20 percent is used for exercise. These relative percentages of energy consumption of course will vary under different circumstances.

When carbohydrates are eaten, about 23 percent of the calories they contain are used to process them. This leaves 77 calories for every 100 carbohydrate calories ingested that can be used by the body. On the other hand, it only takes three calories to turn 100 calories of fat into energy which can be used by the body.[8] Why is there a difference in the efficiency of carbohydrate calories compared to fat calories? It is because the internal thermic loss is greater after eating carbohydrates than after eating a high-fat meal.[9]

Carbohydrates therefore provide fewer net calories available to the body when compared to fats.

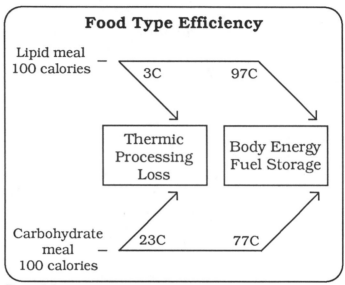

Figure 9-2

Eating fats is like building a home with lumber that has all been precut to size. There will be little waste. Everything ends up in the home. Eating carbohydrates, on the other hand, is like building with boards only one length. Cutting them to size consumes excess energy and creates considerable waste that will not end up in the home structure.

Fats provide about three times the calories of carbohydrates

Conventional nutritional tests list fats as containing approximately nine kilocalories per gram and four for carbohydrates. However, the metabolic differences in the way the body handles fats and carbohydrates, create a difference that is closer to nine for fats and only three for carbohydrates.[10]

Let me explain in a bit more detail why the difference between fat and carbohydrate calories exists. When fats are eaten, their storage requires merely the breakdown of triglycerides, and then their reassembly in adipose tissue. Fat we eat is triglyceride, fat on our body is triglyceride. It's like the precut lumber. (This is not to say the process is simple [see Appendix III, Figure III-1], only that it is efficient.) In contrast, to change the disaccharide carbohydrate sucrose (table sugar) to fat requires its breakdown to the simple sugars glucose and fructose, then conversion to acetyl CoA, reassembly into a fatty acid, then combination with glycerol to form a triglyceride to be stored within adipose tissue. There's a lot of wasted lumber here.[11]

Fat cells are both greedy and stingy

Fat cells are both greedy and stingy. After a meal, fat storage cells eagerly and efficiently take their fill, but then stingily release these fats for oxidation to fulfill the body's energy needs. The body seems to prefer to use energy from carbohydrate, which is stored in the form of glycogen. The formation of glycogen from carbohydrates is an efficient process costing only seven percent of calories ingested, much like the formation of adipose tissue is an efficient process using ingested fats. Carbohydrates are only transformed into fats after body stores of glycogen are filled to their maximum, a feat requiring several days of heavy carbohydrate ingestion.[12]

Glycogen, not fat, is the body's preferred storage form for carbohydrates

But even if glycogen stores were to be filled, and carbohydrate began to form fat, the fat thus formed is thought not to be stored, but instead used for immediate energy needs. It is likely that carbohydrates, therefore, do not directly create adipose tissue. Rather, if taken in sufficient amounts, or in excess, carbohydrates will prevent the oxidation (burning for energy) of fat that is consumed or stored. High carbohydrate consumption, therefore, does not make fat. It simply encourages fat that is consumed to be stored, and fat that is stored to remain there.[13]

It is unlikely that carbohydrates form storage fats

Lipids also stay within their kind in metabolism. That is to say that although consumed, lipids can be oxidized through what is called beta oxidation two carbons at a time to yield energy for the body; they do not convert to carbohydrates. Only the glycerol backbone of triglycerides, which comprises only five percent of triglycerides, can form glucose (see Appendix I). But even this is an inefficient process. The body would rather use ingested carbohydrates to form the glucose for energy needs. Tissues like to store fat for a rainy day.

Lipids like to stay lipids

If carbohydrates are restricted under the belief that by so doing fats will be increasingly oxidized (burnt as body fuel), the results will be disappointing unless fats are also restricted. The body has immediate, and ongoing, needs for blood glucose, but lipids, as mentioned above, are a poor source. The brain is a particular glutton using 60 percent of the glucose used by the entire body in a resting state. When the brain is glucose starved, mood swings occur. In addition, low

Lipids do not form carbohydrates

blood glucose levels from restricted carbohydrate intake can trigger appetite, which can result in hyperphagia (increased food consumption) in an attempt to meet blood glucose needs. The net result may be weight gain rather than loss.

Restricting carbohydrates may in the end result in a net increase in body weight

Organisms are designed to eat natural foods which are inherently balanced with vitamins, minerals, enzymes, fiber, proteins, carbohydrates, and fats. Eaten as such, imbalances such as obesity do not occur. It is only when we are able to strip food fractions out of natural foods, and feed them in disproportionate amounts, that an imbalance such as obesity results. The "calorie is a calorie" myth has done much to foster this food perversion.

The body recognizes increased fat intake as a bounty to be stored

Extracting fats and oils from natural products and then slathering fabricated foods with them to improve mouth feel can result in fat intakes far exceeding those which would be possible in the wild. The body does not recreate the balances that have been lost after foods have been fractionated and fed out of balance. Rather, it performs as it was designed to in a natural setting. In the wild, the body views fats as a prize food material, and stores them with more ease than any other food ingredient. It does not squander the immediate needed energy of carbohydrates by attempting to convert them into fats. Thus, when the body is fed fat, it puts it into reserves, "understanding" that in the wild setting there will be times of feast and famine, and such reserves are necessary for the times of famine. In our lazy, processed-food world, however, these periods of famine come rarely (if ever), which leads to the un-desired and unhealthy building of fat reserves...and obesity.

A variety of other factors can influence the energy availability of foods and their tendency to promote fat deposition and further belie the "calorie is a calorie" myth. The matrix of the food itself can inhibit or enhance the digestion and assimilation process. Processed, refined, fractionated foods are often absorbed rapidly, whereas whole, raw foods create more stool bulk and are absorbed more slowly. The activity of lipoprotein lipase (see Appendix III, p. 244) may vary from individual to individual and affect the deposition of fat in adipose tissue, a factor that again is moderated by a natural food diet. Additionally, saturated fats are deposited in adipose tissue more readily than unsaturated fats.

Unsaturations and their omega position affect caloric value

Additionally — bear with me on this technical stuff for a paragraph — the degree of saturation and the omega position of the first unsaturation, (see Appendix III, p. 245) can affect degree of oxidation. For example, the more highly unsaturated omega -3 fatty acids (e.g. fish, flax, canola oils) and omega -9 oleic fatty acids (e.g. olive oil) are oxidized more readily than are less saturated omega -6 linoleic fatty acids (corn oil, animal fat).[14] The length of the fatty-acid chain can affect caloric efficiency and the tendency toward fat deposition. Long-chain triglycer-

Medium - chain tri- glycerides do not form body fat

ides are readily deposited in fat reserves, whereas medium-chain triglycerides eight to twelve carbons long are not deposited in fat stores, but are readily used for energy by the body.[15] Medium-chain triglycerides are also transported as free fatty acids bound to albumin and moved directly to the liver where they can be oxidized to provide fuel. They can pass into mitochondria (the "power houses" of the cell) and are independent of other biochemicals necessary for the metabolism of long-chain triglycerides, such as carnitine acyltransferase. Additionally, the oxidation of these fatty acids, and the ketones that are a byproduct of their oxidation, provide fuel energy. Medium-chain triglycerides also have an increased thermic effect, which decreases the food energy available for fat deposition. For these reasons, medium-chain triglycerides are a popular food supplement for body builders who need the high energy of fats but desire to look lean and "cut".

Length of fatty acid chain affects caloric value

It becomes apparent from this chapter that weight control is not a matter of mathematics, the simple addition or subtraction of calories. First of all, the caloric value of fatty foods is quite different than previously thought. Their efficient conversion to body fat, particularly as they are presented in processed foods, makes them a far greater culprit than commonly understood. On the other hand, complex carbohydrates provide an excellent fuel source without the fat deposition side effect.

Not all fats are equal either, just as not all calories are equal. The highly unsaturated

*Nutritional
knowledge
is incom-
plete and
so also
will be any
fabricated
food based
on it*

and medium-chain fats found in many fresh vegetables, fruits and wild meat products provide valuable essential health building fatty acids, and they do not contribute to body fat stores. This is why natural high-fat foods such as nuts and avocados are not really fat producing.

From all the rather complex foregoing discussion, we should be led to the inference that foods should be eaten as close to the way they are found in nature as possible. The inherent balances of natural foods help prevent excesses and are in tune with the body's design for food utilization.

We again are led to the wisdom of the Synorgon Diet.

---

1. Wysong, R.L. *The Creation-Evolution Controversy.* Midland, MI: Inquiry Press, 1987.
2. Danforth, Elliot, Jr. "Diet and Obesity." The American Journal of Clinical Nutrition 41 (1985): 1132-1145.
3. Roberts, L. "Diet and health in China." Science 240 (1988): 27.
4. Benum, Sara. "Feast or Famine — An Examination of Weight Management Issues." Complementary Medicine 2 (1987): 10.
5. Oscai, L.B., et al. "Effect of dietary fat on food intake, growth and body composition in rats." Growth 48 (1984): 415-424.
6. Benum, Sara. "Feast or Famine — An Examination of Weight Management Issues." Complementary Medicine 2 (1987): 10.
7. Pi-Sunyer, F. Xavier. "Obesity" in *Modern Nutrition in Health and Disease.* Philadelphia: Lea & Febiger, 1988, p. 804.
8. Journal of Clinical Nutrition 76 (1985): 1019.
8a. American Journal of Physiology 246 (1984): E62.
8b. Metabolism 31 (1982): 1234.
9. Danforth, Elliot, Jr. "Diet and Obesity." The American Journal of Clinical Nutrition 41 (1985): 1132-1145.

10. Rolfes, Sharon Rady, M.S., R.D. "A Matter of Fat." Nutrition Clinics 5, No. 3 (May/June, 1990): 5-6.

10a. Petosa, R. "Self-actualization and health related practices." Health Education (May/June 1984): 9-12.

11. Danforth, E. "Diet and obesity." The American Journal of Clinical Nutrition 41 (1985):1132-1145.

11a. Leveille, G.A., et al. "Isocaloric diets: Effects of dietary changes." The American Journal of Clinical Nutrition 45 (1987): 158-163.

12. Acheson, K.J., et al. "Glycogen storage capacity and de novo lipogenesis during massive carbohydrate overfeeding in man." The American Journal of Clinical Nutrition 48 (1988): 240-247.

13. Flatt, J.P. "Effect of carbohydrate and fat intake on postprandial substrate oxidation and storage." Topics in Clinical Nutrition 2 (1987): 15-27.

14. Storlien, L.H. "Not all dietary fats may lead to obesity." The American Journal of Clinical Nutrition 51 (1990): 1114.

15. Senior, J.R. Introductory remarks by Chairman. In *Medium Chain Triglycerides.* Philadelphia: University of Pennsylvania Press, 1968.

15a. Hashim, S.A. "Studies of medium chain fatty acid transport in portal blood" in *Medium Chain Triglycerides.* Philadelphia: University of Pennsylvania Press, 1968.

15b. Fiaccadori, F., et al. "Branched chain amino acid enriched solutions in the treatment of hepatic encephalopathy in a controlled trial." in *Hepatic Encephalopathy in Chronic Liver Failure.* New York: Plenum Publishing Corp., 1984, pp. 323-333.

10 - GENETICS

To what degree is obesity genetically determined and beyond our control?

Evidence demonstrating a genetic influence includes studies showing that adoptees follow the weight patterns of their natural parents rather than that of their adoptive parents.[1] Identical twins, widely separated environmentally, may also show very similar weight management problems.[2,3]

Adoptees follow the weight of their natural parents

Although no specific genetic marker has been found, phenotypically (the outward physical manifestation of genes) the defect is expressed through decreased thermogenesis (energy expenditure).[4] Decreased thermogenesis translates into increased body fat deposition.[5]

Some evidence argues that it is thinness that has a genetic component, rather than obesity. Thus it may be improperly functioning "thinness genes" that are responsible for obesity, rather than an "obesity gene" per se.[6,7] The genetic defect may therefore be one of omission rather than commission, so to speak.

Specific genetically controlled metabolic factors which could lead to obesity include disturbances in thyroid and other hormones; neuropeptide (brain chemical) imbalance; low levels of epidermal growth factor; and increased levels of galanin — a brain chemical which can increase fat craving.[8,9]

70

Having a genetic weakness, however, does not mean the weakness must surface. Stress (environmental, emotional, physical) is what causes genetic defects to be manifest. Given any stress, some individuals within a population will suffer more than others. Even highly lethal epidemics affect only a portion of the population, with some maintaining their health unscathed.

Appetite and satiety are innate mechanisms capable of assuring survival in the wild

We are all genetically and biochemically highly individualistic. Subtle biochemical genetic weaknesses may never even be noticed until the right kind of challenge occurs. For example, running speed is unimportant to survival unless attempting to avoid a car or a predator. In a group attempting to escape, those with the genetic "defect" for slowness would most likely be injured. In the "race" for healthy weight, those with the genetic weakness for high fats, refined foods, and sedentary living fall victim. The genetic inclination to obesity would likely not, therefore, be given opportunity to express itself given the conditions in the wild.

Like a plague, obesity follows modern living around the world. Indigenous "wild" cultures are obesity-free until we set up our burger and fry stands and wean these poor "undeveloped" people onto baby formula, Coke and Twinkies. The Pima Indians of Southeastern Arizona are an excellent case in point. Modern living has christened them with an exceptionally high incidence of obesity and the highest level of adult onset diabetes in the world. There is nothing really wrong with their genetics. Rather, the fault lies in their new modern way of life.[10]

The genetic component of obesity is not a defect at all except within the context of our modern, altered conditions of food abundance, food fractions, and excess leisure. Similarly, two workers may work in a modern factory that generates high levels of dust and pollutants within the workplace air. One may succumb to emphysema or even cancer, and the other may work at his shoulder on to retirement with never a health problem. The worker falling to disease under these conditions is not defective genetically, but simply genetically more susceptible to this form of stress. If this unusual stress were not present, the worker would never have had the disease.

It seems reasonable to predict that the vast majority of obesity cases could be prevented or reversed by eliminating the conditions which create the "stress" and set the stage for imbalance. Even given an extreme genetic predisposition toward obesity, such individuals forced to obtain their food by foraging in the wild on a daily basis would simply not be capable of building the prodigious bulk that some individuals are able to in our modern setting. First, natural raw foods would never be in such abundance as to permit long-term over-consumption; second, in order to obtain foods, sometimes vast amounts of energy would have to be expended; and third, if weight were somehow accumulated in excess, survival itself would be threatened, because it would not be possible to perform the daily tasks necessary for survival.

The modern world permits the genetic expression of obesity

The wild would not permit obesity

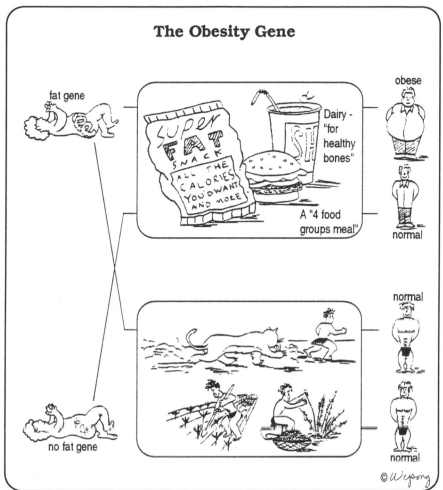

Figure 10-1

The genetic inclination toward obesity is not an unalterable fate. It is also not a valid excuse for those wanting to play victim rather than take control of life.

There is hope regardless of the genetic hand we have been dealt. We must reestablish "wild" synorgonic lifestyle and eating patterns. By so doing, we inhibit the expression of obesity genes. In a later chapter, I will specifically outline how this can easily be accomplished.

---

1. Stunkard, A.J., et al. "A Twin Study of Human Obesity." The Journal of the American Medical Association 256 (1986): 51-54.
2. Shields, J. *Monozygotic Twins Brought up Apart and Brought up Together.* London: Oxford University Press, 1962.
2a. Newman, H.H., et al. *Twins: A Study of Heredity and Environment.* Chicago: University of Chicago Press, 1937.
3. Ravussin, Eric, and Swinburn, Boyd A. "Pathophysiology of Obesity." The Lancet 340 (1992): 404.
4. Surgical Management of Morbid Obesity (Science and Practice of Surgery[12].) Ed. Ward O. Griffin, Jr., and Kenneth J. Printen. New York: Marcek Dekker, 1987.
5. Roberts, Susan B., et al. "Energy Expenditure and Intake in Infants Born to Lean and Overweight Mothers." The New England Journal of Medicine 318 (1988): 461.
6. Weiss, S.R., "Obesity, Pathogenesis, Consequences, and Approaches to Treatment." Psychiatric Clinics of North America 7 (1984): 307-319.
6a. Stunkard, A.J., et al. "A Twin Study of Human Obesity." The Journal of the American Medical Association 256 (1986): 51-54.
6b. Stunkard, A.J., et al. "An Adoption Study of Human Obesity." New England Journal of Medicine 314 (1986): 193-198.
7. Constanzo, P.R., and Schiffman, S.S. "Thinness – Not Obesity – Has a Genetic Component." Neuroscience & Biobehavioral Reviews 13 (1): 55-58.
8. Lauer, Michael S., M.D., et al. "The Impact of Obesity on Left Ventricular Mass and Geometry." The Journal of the American Medical Association 266 (1991): 231.
9. Ezzel, C. "Craving fat? Blame it on a Brain Protein." Science News 142 (1992): 311.
10. Knowler, W.C., et al. "Diabetes Incidence in Pima Indians: Contribution of Obesity and Parental Diabetes." Americal Journal of Epidemiology 113 (1981): 144-56.

Aside from genetics, other powerful physical pulls lead us to obesity. The modern lifestyle and modern processed diet can actually turn us into drug addicts. Not the criminal kind, but a more insidious, socially accepted kind that can destroy health and life just as surely. Here's how.

All life is addicted to its food. Eating brings pleasure, comfort, and satiety, and keeps us coming back for more. Other necessities, such as breathing, sleeping and elimination, could likewise be called addicting. They are metabolically necessary for survival, and are thus intimately linked to pleasure centers in the brain to ensure that what is necessary for survival is done on a continuing basis.

Addiction to the pleasures derived from many of life's functions is essential to survival

These essentially involuntary functions have their roots deep within our neural and endocrine (hormone) systems. Pain, pleasure, delight, love, and hate are rewards and consequences that force an organism to do that which promotes survival and to avoid that which threatens it. Thus, eating, breathing, seeking shelter, reproducing, and eliminating are pleasurable. Not being able to do these things brings unpleasantness, if not outright pain.

The pleasure and pain centers located in what is called the limbic primitive core of the brain, provide the proper motivation for the higher centers in the cortex (grey matter) to make choices that result in more pleasure than pain, and thus a greater chance for survival. These pleasure and pain centers are perfect for organisms within a natural environment. However, we have now been radically extracted from that environment and have surrounded ourselves with a glut of sensory possibilities that are not related to survival, but which can nevertheless arouse pleasure centers. The resulting imbalance from the continual abuse of these pleasure centers can create obesity and resultant health damage.

Abuse of pleasure centers meant for survival is the root of addiction

Bear with me now as I indulge in some detail to help you understand the link between obesity and addiction. Once you understand it, you will also see how to "break the habit" and begin a new life of health and vitality.

The autonomic nervous system governs those things outside of our direct volitional control. It consists of two parts. First, the parasympathetic system governs actions such as sleeping, eating, elimination, and other organ metabolic functions primarily having to do with maintenance and restoration.

The second part is the sympathetic nervous system — the "fight or flight" controller. The sympathetic system is arousing in nature and prepares us for adjusting to and mastering our environment. It promotes curiosity, creativity, and challenge, and can also bring pleasure.

The sympathetic system functions through the neurotransmitter dopamine. Dopamine stimulates pleasure in the limbic system within the brain. On the other hand, the parasympathetic system is stimulated to pleasure by the neurotransmitter chemicals known as endorphins.

Thus, both parts of the autonomic nervous system can bring us pleasure: the parasympathetic through "lower" fundamental biological functions such as eating; the other, sympathetic, through "higher" functions such as problem solving.

Balancing pleasures derived from sympathetic and parasympathetic systems is a key to health

The parasympathetic system is more fully developed and active in infancy than the sympathetic system. Certain aspects of the sympathetic system, such as exploring, curiosity, creativity, and otherwise gaining pleasure from an aroused state, are learned and require time and input from the higher brain centers. When we are born we need basic metabolic functions fully formed but do not yet need to contemplate $E=MC^2$. Our parents take care of these higher mental functions for us. But we do need to let them know when we're hungry, full, or need our diaper changed. Thus we are parasympathetic (endorphin) addicts in infancy.

A balanced, happy, adjusted, and productive adult life, however, is one that derives pleasure from both systems. There is pleasure from the aroused sympathetic state through exercise, recreation, and the challenge of work. Pleasure from the recuperative parasympathetic stage requires eating and resting.

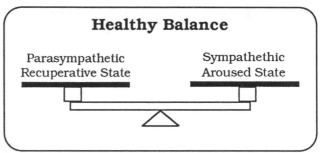

Figure 11-1

Challenge, balanced with recuperative rest, is what our very being longs for

If for one reason or another an organism becomes imbalanced, such that more emphasis is placed on the parasympathetic system with eating and resting predominating, the result can be depression from excess parasympathetic chemicals. Depression can then lead to further inactivity and overeating, and the cycle escalates. On the other side, overstimulation of the sympathetic system can result in psychotic disturbances, nervousness, and anxiety from oversecretion of sympathetic chemicals.

A life filled with days of creative, exciting challenge, balanced with healthful food and recuperative rest, is what our very being longs for. It is this balance that should be sought as a necessary ingredient to health and happiness, not the one-sided pleasures from an emphasis on one system or the other.

Knowledge of the various chemical mediators of the autonomic nervous system has led to the production of a variety of pharma-

ceuticals as well as street drugs. But, when
we start chemically manipulating this complex internal biochemistry, watch out.

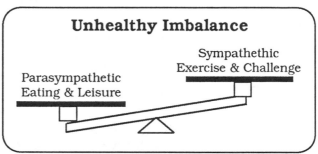

Unhealthy Imbalance

Parasympathetic
Eating & Leisure

Sympathethic
Exercise & Challenge

Figure 11-2

***Drugs can
abuse
survival
pleasure
centers***

Severe imbalance is possible through the
use of pharmaceuticals such as amphetamines, cocaine, morphine, methadone, alcohol, and nicotine. Some such chemicals
can stimulate the release of dopamine within
the limbic system. Thus, an internal pleasure chemical such as dopamine, which is
supposed to result from healthful living activities, is now stimulated without requiring
those activities. Other chemicals, such as
heroin, can mimic the endorphin parasympathetic system, creating pleasure without
the appropriate recuperative balancing activities meant to create these pleasures. This
is the root of drug addiction. We simply cheat
our bodies by getting pleasure without doing
the healthful things such pleasure is meant
to ensure.

Some exogenous (from the outside) chemicals are capable of stimulating the release of
the body's own endorphins and dopamines,
while others may simply mimic these chemicals and compete with the body's biochemi-

cals for receptor sites on neurons. Morphine, for example, competes with endorphins for their receptor sites.

Food tolerance is like drug tolerance

When drug abuse occurs, the body does not sit by passively. It reacts to the over-abundance of dopamine stimulants, or endorphin stimulants, by decreasing its own production of these chemicals in an effort to achieve balance. This is called negative feedback. Then if the drugs are withdrawn, the body is unable to gain pleasure from normal sympathetic and parasympathetic activities, because of insufficient output of these neurotransmitters. The pleasure centers become dependent upon exogenous input. Thus is born drug dependence.

Drugs replace survival actions in producing pleasure

As more drugs are taken, less endogenous transmitters are manufactured. Normal living creates less and less pleasure and dependence deepens. Tolerance then increases, requiring more and more of the chemical to get the same effect. When withdrawal from the exogenous drug occurs, the body is left without any pleasure-stimulating chemicals. The pain of withdrawal can become excruciating until the body reinvigorates its own pleasure-producing chemical system.

Drugs can mimic survival mechanisms

Repeatedly taking drugs, or other addictive substances, perverts the body's pleasure-driven health and survival centers. Pleasure, then, seeks an appetite for itself, unrelated to important survival activities. The drive for stimulation becomes so overpowering that animals and humans have been known to seek the stimulation from these endocrine pleasure chemicals by choosing substances such as sugar and addictive drugs over nourishing food to the point of starvation and death.

Virtually any substance or activity can be addictive

Not every organism is equally susceptible to these imbalances. Biochemical individuality ranges from the highly resistant to the easily addicted personality. Here again is that individualized genetic factor discussed in the previous chapter.

Often, substance abuse simply follows various other addictive behaviors as a pattern throughout life. Addiction is not restricted to simply that which is illegal. Workaholics, exerciseaholics, sugarholics, chocolateholics, coffeeholics, cigarretteholics, all are moved by similar stimulatory mecha-

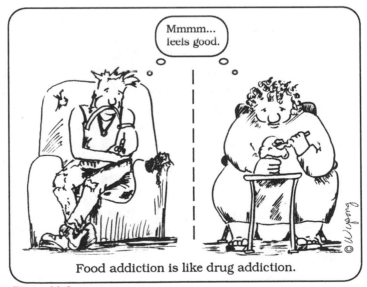

Food addiction is like drug addiction.

Figure 11-3

nisms, and often those who do one also do others as a part of their addictive personality.

Now how does this more specifically relate to food and obesity? Eating, both in terms of how much we eat and what kinds of food we select, can indeed be addicting. Survival pleasure centers in the brain can be stimulated to crave foods that are unhealthy.

Addictive behavior comes in groups

Many lines of evidence support the view that eating disorders can parallel substance abuse, both in terms of the impact on the individual, and in terms of biochemistry. Figure 11-4 shows, for example, the nutrient precursors (chemical building blocks) required for various neurotransmitters in the brain. If these neurotransmitters exist in excess, or in deficiency, imbalances leading to aberrant behaviors may occur, including anorexia nervosa, bulimia, overeating, and overconsumption of certain foods.

Eating stimulates the parasympathetic system, releasing pleasurable endorphins. These are opiates, which have been found to be blocked by the same opiate antagonists (such as naloxone) that can block the opium used by a drug addict. This is proof that the same mechanisms at work in eating disorders are also at work in chemical addictions. It is also interesting to note that naloxone can even block the enjoyment of music. This demonstrates that endorphins are likely also responsible for the pleasure we receive from this activity, and thus even music may be addicting.

Some Neurotransmitters, Their Functions, And The Nutrient Precursors

Neurotransmitter	Functions and Nutrient Precursors
Acetylcholine	Inhibits involuntary functions, such as heart rate; works in nerve-muscle connections and in the cerebral cortex, the brain area responsible for reasoning, thought, and memory. Abnormalities in these areas cause Alzheimer's disease. Made from choline, a widely distributed food component.
Dopamine	Regulates motor activity and helps brain discriminate reality from fantasy; destruction of these brain parts results in Parkinson's disease. Made from the amino acid tyrosine.
Endorphins	Act on the brain's opiate receptors to inhibit pain and cause sedation; also called endogenous opiates, or enkephalins. Made from dietary amino acids.
GABA (Gamma-aminobutyric acid)	Inhibits action of the brain's cortex and affects more brain neurons than any other single neurotransmitter. Made from the amino acid glutamate.
Norepinephrine	Excites neurons responsible for stress response (accelerated heartbeat, elevated blood pressure, increased muscle tension.) Made from dopamine, and therefore depends on the amino acid tyrosine.
Serotonin	Inhibits action of the brain stem, regulates sleep and relaxation. Abnormalities associated with mood disorders, such as manic-depressive disorder. Made from the amino acid tryptophan, whose transport into the brain is enhanced by the presence of carbohydrate.

Figure 11-4

Further evidencing the link between eating disorders, obesity, and drug addiction, blood levels of beta endorphins have been found to be higher in the obese. Opioid agonists (promoters), such as methadone and butorphanol tartrate will stimlulate food intake because they enhance the activities of these parasympathetic endorphins.

Eating disorders and obesity are linked to powerful, deep-seated biochemical mechanisms and resultant, almost involuntary, Pavlovian pleasure seeking pulls. This helps us to realize that such addictive problems are not just a matter of will, stubbornness, depravity, and the like.

"Drug" abuse is possible without ever taking drugs

Addictions to the eating parasympathetic pulls can be overcome by restoring appropriate balances and particularly by increasing the rewards and pleasures we receive from the sympathetic system through exercise, challenging work, overcoming helplessness, creativity, exploiting our curiosity, and doing good. These are much better and healthier anorexics than any drug.

Unfortunately, attaining balance can be difficult in our modern society of readily available substances that can be abused. These substances include chemicals and food — particularly processed fractionated foods which, in their isolated new chemical forms, are very much like drugs.

Much can be done to not only prevent, but to treat, food addictions and their resulting unhealthy balances. We can move the diet to fresh, whole, raw, natural foods as much as possible; make fun forms of exercise a part of everyday life; and seek challenging, creative, worthwhile work (sympathetic) along with appropriate, enjoyable leisure and rest (parasympathetic).

The neurotransmitter view of substance abuse and food imbalances provides a very rational understanding of why we act as we do. We tend to think that the choices we make in life are a matter of our will, our abstract volitional being, rather than a result of pulls and pressures from more intrinsic biochemical and physiological mechanisms. Increasing evidence shows that much of what we do is a result of the pleasure or pain we feel from doing it.

Abuse of food or leisure was not an option in the wild

It makes sense that such a mechanism would influence our choices. Nature has not left us to our unpredictable, free will to decide if or when to do things that are essential to our survival. Within the primitive core of our brain are mechanisms to draw us to, or push us away from acts, depending upon whether these acts contribute or take away from survivability.

In the wild it is likely that innate biological mechanisms would work very well for us. In fact, we can be assured they did. Otherwise we would not exist today. In the wild there would be little opportunity for excesses. Sleeping and eating endorphin pleasures would likely follow productive, challenging, creative activity finding food and maintaining shelter — dopamine pleasures. One without the other was not even a choice.

Coddled living and unlimited foods are powerful drugs

But today we are surrounded by almost unlimited options. The ability to have food always readily available, the ability to be coddled by jobs that require little from us other than our presence from nine to five, with wages perhaps out of balance with the worth of our activities, and benefits and vacation prenegotiated for us by a society bent on ease, makes it easy for us to stimulate pleasure centers that were meant to be stimulated by activities which enhance health and survivability.

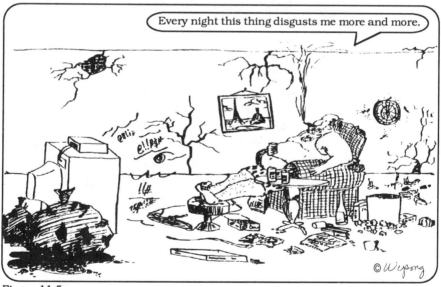

Figure 11-5

In other words, we are in the position of being able to artificially derive pleasure from the parasympathetic endorphin chemicals that are meant to assure appropriate rest and nutrition. We vegetate in front of a television for hours on end, or sit at our work rather than engage in active, manual activities. We sleep in and have available to us virtually unlimited supplies of food in any form we desire. We are like children with unlimited money turned loosed in a candy store, like a fox with free access to a hen house, or like a rutting bull with access to an entire herd of bovine damsels in peak estrus. The opportunity for glut, and thus imbalance and damage, is exceptionally rare, if not nonexistent, in the wild. But today we are faced with the opportunity to stimulate our pleasure systems with abandon.

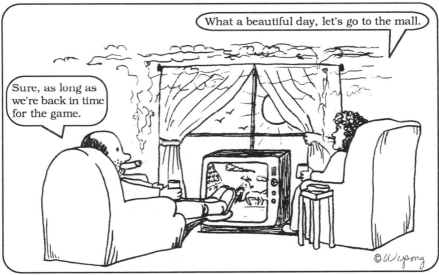

Figure 11-6

If we recognize that by stimulating one center or the other disproportionately on a repeated basis, that we can become addicted to the pleasures derived therefrom, we can be more cautious and also understand the need to invoke the higher centers of our brain, to override the pull of these pleasure centers.

Children have choices made for them. Most parents do not allow children to squander away days simply lollygagging on the couch. Nor do they allow free access to candy on a continuing basis. If they did, higher, yet undeveloped sympathetically oriented centers would easily be overcome by gluttony in one form or another. Sickness and disease would surely follow such imbalanced activity.

As adults, we have the opportunity to indulge without limit. We must use the same intellect that creates our modern, artificial society of imbalance and excess to achieve moderation and balance. This does not mean denial. Rather, it can mean fuller pleasures from living life in balance and enjoying the spectrum of life's stimulating activities. Health, vitality, and maintaining appropriate weight are of course an added bonus.[1-5]

---

1. Rogers, R.J. *Endorphins, Opiates, and Behavioral Processes.* New York: John Wiley & Sons, 1988.
2. Fullerton, D.T., et al. "Sugar, Opioids, and Binge Eating." Brain Research Bulletin 14 (June 1985): 673-680.
3. Olson, G.A., et al. "Endogenous Opiates: 1983." Peptides 5 (1984): 179.
4. Black, Dean, Ph.D. "Addictions, Why They Enslave Us, How to Break Free." The Healing Currents Series (1989): 1-16.
5. Sizer, Francis. "Addiction, Brain Chemistry, and Eating Disorders." Nutrition Clinics, Vol. 4, No. 2 (March/April, 1989): 1-16.

12 - FOOD & MOOD

An imbalance in life, including food excess, can dramatically impact our pleasure and pain centers and make us addicted slaves to unhealthy living patterns. We can be led through life by our tongue and dig our grave with our teeth.

Modern living can also cause addiction to certain food substances. This is a result of a weakened immune system and an unnaturally altered food supply. The foods we are addicted to may even be the foods we are allergic to. But this, yet another health-robbing consequence of modern life, is the topic of another book someday.

Processed carbohy-drates toy with the mood elevator serotonin

In this chapter, I want to briefly discuss how our mood, our very ability to enjoy life, is directly affected by the character of the food we eat. Obese individuals often describe how depression drives them not only to eating excesses, but to junk food orgies. Here's why.

Another neurochemical affecting mood and appetite that is influenced by the food we eat is serotonin.

Serotonin promotes sleep and relaxation and can, if deficient, cause depression. Pharmacologic antidepressants, in fact, often work by increasing the action of serotonin.

Biochemical mediators that control appetite are ancient and pervasive throughout the biological world. Even a creature as primitive as the leech produces serotonin (from the Retzius cells in the subesophageal ganglia — in case you wanted to know!) which controls appetite and satiety analogously to its action in humans.[1] Our link with nature is intricate and inextricable.

The level of serotonin in the brain is indirectly linked to carbohydrate consumption by the following mechanism. Serotonin

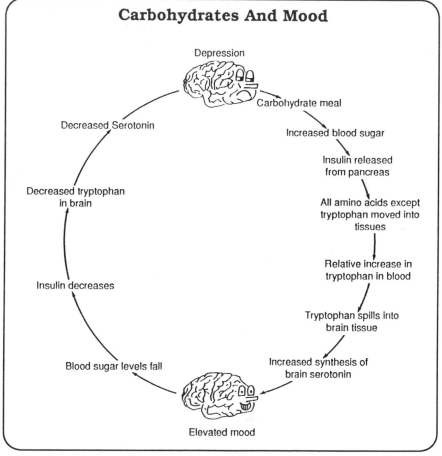

Carbohydrates And Mood

Depression

Carbohydrate meal

Decreased Serotonin

Increased blood sugar

Insulin released
from pancreas

Decreased tryptophan
in brain

All amino acids except
tryptophan moved into
tissues

Relative increase in
tryptophan in blood

Insulin decreases

Tryptophan spills into
brain tissue

Blood sugar levels fall

Increased synthesis of
brain serotonin

Elevated mood

Figure 12-1

is synthesized from the amino acid (a building block of protein) tryptophan. So if more tryptophan can move into the brain from the blood vessels, more serotonin will be produced and mood will be lifted. By an interesting mechanism, the ingestion of carbohydrates does this.

Refined carbohydrate consumption can be directly related to mood

When carbohydrates are eaten, the body releases insulin that not only moves the carbohydrates into cells for fuel, but also moves amino acids into cells as well. But insulin preferentially pulls more of all amino acids from the blood into muscle and other tissues than tryptophan, leaving a relative abundance of this amino acid in the blood after a carbohydrate meal. The relative high blood level of tryptophan then "spills" into brain tissue, resulting in serotonin production and elevated mood.

Refined processed carbohydrates (sugar, white flour) stimulate peaks in blood sugar followed by a rapid release of insulin, which then drops blood sugar levels to below normal. After these levels drop, tryptophan must compete with other amino acids to enter the brain, and thus serotonin is lowered below the threshold necessary for stabilization of mood. Depression results, often provoking another refined carbohydrate meal. When this occurs, blood sugar peaks, insulin is squeezed from the pancreas, tryptophan increases and moves into the brain to again produce serotonin, and mood is elevated.

The effect of processed carbohydrate meals on children is often particularly evident as they alternate between climbing the walls and being sullen, cranky monsters. It's thus easy to be left with the mistaken impression that such meals are the way to feel good.

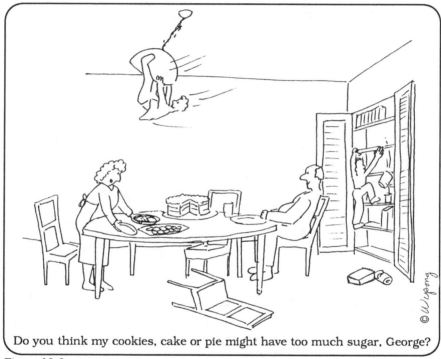

Do you think my cookies, cake or pie might have too much sugar, George?

Figure 12-2

Thus our quest to simply feel good results in an escalating cycle of refined carbohydrate binges. The end result of this cycle is disease from the secondary effects of the resulting obesity, pancreatic stress, and diabetes.

It is by manipulating these various neurotransmitter mechanisms that anorexic drugs exert their effect. For example, monoamine oxidase inhibitors depress the appetite because monoamine oxidase is responsible for breaking down serotonin. Thus if less serotonin is broken down, its levels remain higher, mood remains lifted, and the craving for carbohydrate decreases. Amphetamine, phenylpropanolamine, and fenfluramine are also drugs which act on serotonin, as do the neurochemicals dopamine and noradrenalin.

The best anorexic is a balanced life

Such pharmacologic intervention is only needed due to the imbalances modern living has created in physiological systems that are designed to help us survive, be healthy, and be happy. Far better it is to address causes rather than attempt to force the body into compliance with a synthetic chemical arsenal.

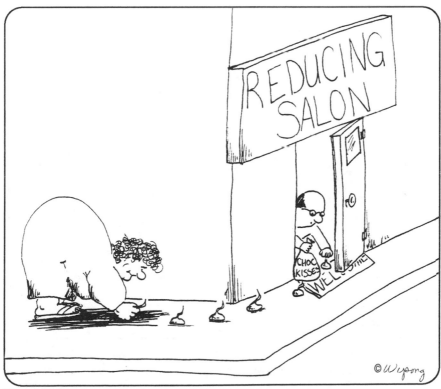

Figure 12-3

The Glycemic Index of Common Foods

Grain, cereal products

Buckwheat	51 ±	10
Bread (white)	69 ±	5
Bread (whole meal)	72 ±	6
Millet	71 ±	10
Pastry	59 ±	6
Rice (brown)	66 ±	5
Rice (white)	72 ±	9
Spaghetti (whole meal)	42 ±	4
Spaghetti (white)	50 ±	8
Sponge cake	46 ±	6
Sweet corn	59 ±	11

Breakfast cereals

All-bran	52 ±	5
Cornflakes	80 ±	6
Meusli	66 ±	9
Porridge oats	49 ±	8
Shredded wheat	67 ±	10
Wheatabix	75 ±	10

Biscuits

Digestive	59 ±	7
Oatmeal	54 ±	4
Rich tea	55 ±	4
Ryvita	69 ±	10

Dried legumes

Beans (tinned, baked)	40 ±	3
Beans (butter)	36 ±	4
Beans (haricot)	31 ±	6
Beans (kidney)	29 ±	8
Beans (soya)	15 ±	5
Beans (tinned, soya)	14 ±	2
Peas (blackeye)	33 ±	4
Peas (chick)	36 ±	5
Peas (marrowfat)	47 ±	3
Lentils	29 ±	3

Dairy products

Ice cream	36 ±	8
Milk (skim)	32 ±	5
Milk (whole)	34 ±	6
Yogurt	36 ±	4

Vegetables

Broad beans	79 ±	16
Frozen peas	51 ±	6

Root vegetables

Beetroot	64 ±	16
Carrots	92 ±	20
Parsnips	97 ±	19
Potato (instant)	80 ±	13
Potato (new)	70 ±	8
Potato (sweet)	48 ±	6
Swede	72 ±	8
Yam	51 ±	12

Fruit

Apples (gold. del.)	39 ±	3
Banana	62 ±	9
Oranges	40 ±	3
Orange juice	46 ±	6
Raisins	64 ±	11

Sugars

Fructose	20 ±	5
Glucose	100 ±	
Maltose	105 ±	12
Sucrose	59 ±	10

Miscellaneous

Fish fingers	38 ±	6
Honey	87 ±	8
Lucozade	95 ±	10
Mars bar	68 ±	12
Peanuts	13 ±	6
Potato crisps	51 ±	7
Sausages	28 ±	6
Tomato soup	38 ±	9

Foods with the highest numbers cause the highest and most rapid rise in blood sugar.

From The American Journal of Clinical Nutrition 34 (1981): 363.

Figure 12-4

Serotonin-related mood swings ultimately result from surges and depletions of blood sugars (carbohydrates). Refined sugars and flours cause rapid rises in blood sugars, whereas whole natural foods slowly release their sugars to the blood.

Food scientists have ranked foods according to their ability to cause rapid blood sugar increases. Those highest in this glycemic index cause the most elevation in blood sugar following meals. Notice in Figure 12-4 that those with the highest number on the list are generally refined, highly processed foods, while those with lower numbers are more natural and whole in character.

If more natural whole foods are consumed in place of high-glycemic foods, radical mood swings are replaced with a more sustained positive mood, due to the more even release of sugars and serotonin.

This complex serotonin-insulin-amino acid mechanism is used by medicine as a clue for the synthesis of potential drugs. Food scientists, on the other hand, simply rank fabricated foods on a glycemic index chart. Both miss the obvious: we have removed ourselves from our natural whole food synorgonic context. Sustained health will only be restored when we return as much as possible to this context.

---

1. Blundell, John E. "Serotonin and the biology of feeding." The American Journal of Clinical Nutrition 55S (1992): 155.

13 - APPETITE

Eating by the clock can override innate weight control mechanisms

Appetite is part biological, part social and part conditioned. How do we control our appetite? It is a consequence of a complex set of dynamic factors, and not simply a timed mechanism such as the daily sleep and wake cycle. Healthy appetite mechanisms become obscured, distorted, and arguably perverted by the availability of irresistable-tasting food at arm's length almost any time of the day. Our innate controls are also confused by a kaleidoscope of compelling flavor options, and daily schedules which dictate eating by the clock ("It's suppertime, I must be hungry"), rather than by physiological need.

In the wild, appetite is an essential component of survival. Organisms are keenly tuned to the complex feedback mechanisms that exist between the digestive tract, organs, endocrine system, brain, and neurotransmitters. These all interplay to tell the organism when, how much, and even what to eat in order to best survive.

Appetite is capable of guiding balanced eating

Hunger and satiety are regulated by sugar, insulin, and amino acid blood levels; fat stores; digestive hormones such as cholecystokinin; and a broad range of other chemicals that dictate when enough is enough, and when more is needed.[1]

The appetite mechanism is located in the hypothalamus, a more primitive part of the brain stem.[2] A meal containing high levels of carbohydrates results in signals to the hypothalmus stimulating an appetite for increased protein at the next meal. Pregnancy, with its extraordinary demands, gives a glimpse of what inherent taste/survival capabilities lie within us. Pregnancy can result in exaggeration of these mechanisms with an increased taste for salt, resulting in midnight raids for pickles and anchovies. Even pica, such as the eating of dirt, during pregnancy may reflect a need for calcium or other minerals.[3]

Natural appetite encourages food variety

The appetite is designed to cause the consumption of a variety of foods. If a single food is eaten, there soon will follow a decreased appetite for that food. For example, if before eating candy one were to consume sugar, the appetite for the candy would dramatically fall. This is the rationale for single food type diets. By consuming only one food, such as grapefruits, appetite for carbohydrates can theoretically be decreased.[4]

Single food tolerance is similar to drug tolerance

Tolerance for certain foods can be increased with repeated consumption. For example, if a diet high in sweets is continually eaten, more sweets are required to obtain the same satisfaction. This, as we have discussed previously, relates closely to other forms of drug addiction, where tolerance to the drug over time increases, so that more and more is required for the same measure of satisfaction. Reprogramming the senses can be done either through gradual reduction in the food type that is being consumed in excess, or eliminating it entirely for a period of time.

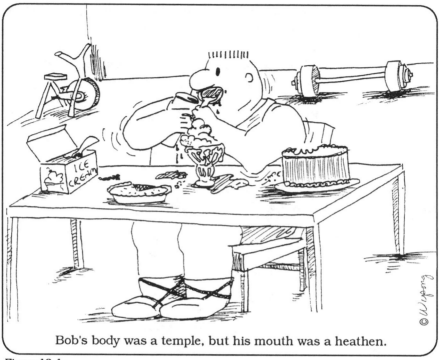

Bob's body was a temple, but his mouth was a heathen.

Figure 13-1

The presence of the "on" eating switch, in combination with continual food abundance, is a genetic anachronism

There is also an on and off switch for eating. Usually when one begins eating, provided the food tastes good, eating is continued until satiety is reached. "On" eating mechanisms make it difficult for one to simply begin eating, and then stop. That's why the challenge "I bet you can't eat just one" works.

This mechanism is designed for our natural setting — that is, the wild. In the wild, where food is scarce and abundance occasional, the body is programmed to eat to satisfaction when opportunity presents itself. In the wild, if a carnivore spent a week without food, finally killed prey, but only consumed two mouthfuls, got bored and left the remains to scavengers, it is not likely the carnivore would live long. Instead, when a kill is made, the carnivore eats to capacity, and may do so over a period of days, gorging itself until the prey is either entirely eaten or stolen by other animals. After the animal is full, it is content and does not expend the often incredible energy necessary to pursue more prey.

The same brain that can trick the palate, and create unnaturally abundant supplies of food, must be used to moderate instinctual urges designed for a wild setting

Similarly, people in the wild who happen upon a marsh of plentiful berries would not be wise to simply eat a few mouthfuls and then move on to what might be several days' travel before more food is available. There is great satisfaction in eating to capacity. The body is concerned that it be full at every opportunity in a natural world, where the pursuit of food could require almost every waking hour.

The body did not, however, expect the abundance of modern society. In our present setting, food is readily available almost any time. Pantries bulge, refrigerators are heaped, restaurants beckon on every corner, and we feel guilty if the pet's bowl is ever empty. When we begin to eat, our eating switch is turned on and we usually eat to capacity, as if we had just captured our prey. This can happen several times a day rather than the once or twice a day or every few days that would likely be more natural, healthy, and possible in the natural setting. Thus, the "on" eating switch may be, in fact, a genetic defect in our modern setting. This is yet more proof that we are in a genetic time warp.

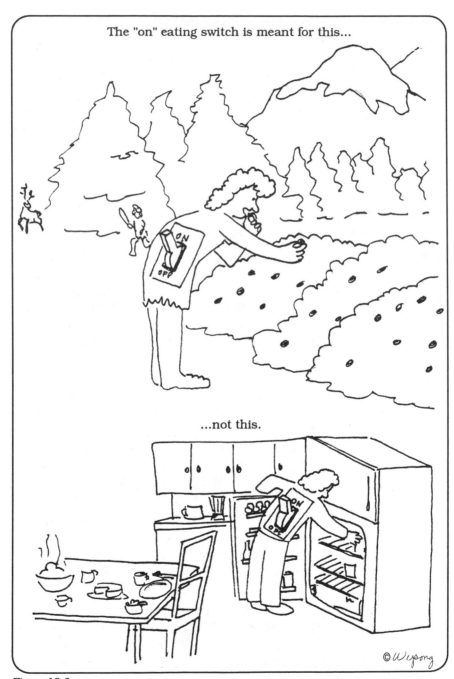

Figure 13-2

By understanding that we are physiologically under the powerful influences of "on" eating switches, and that modern commerical food enterprises have made a sophisticated art and science of leading us around by the tongue, we must be wary and use the same brain which created such circumstances to tell us how to control, moderate, and stop. Being aware that if we begin to eat, that powerful biological mechanisms are triggered to keep us eating, provides valuable insight as to how to control food intake.

---

1. Hirsch, Cheryl. "Appetite Control." Medical Nutrition, Vol. 5, No. 2, (Winter 1990): 32.
2. Ibid. 33.
3. Bland, Jeffrey S., Ph.D. "Weight Management and its Relationship to Hunger, Appetite and Satiety — Is Food Preference Related to Nutrient Need?" Complementary Medicine, Vol. 2, No. 3, (Jan./Feb. 1987): 6.
4. Ibid.

14 - EXERCISE

Let's begin this chapter by putting to rest two serious misconceptions regarding exercise and weight control. The first one goes something like this. In order for you to lose one pound of fat, you must walk 30 miles or play the equivalent of 11 hours of volleyball. Such depressing statistics are enough to make anyone quit before starting. Weight control is not a mathematical problem solved in a laboratory. Measuring a food's caloric content in a bomb calorimeter, then measuring how many calories are burned in exercise, and making a simple subtraction will not determine whether weight will be gained or lost. As we have previously described, weight is neither added nor subtracted by such measures. A food's biological caloric value simply cannot be determined by incinerating it in a laboratory.

There are many uncertainties about how to control weight, but there is no uncertainty as to whether exercise can reduce weight. It is very simple. In order for us to live, even lying in bed in deep REM sleep, energy is required. That energy is derived from the foods we eat. The more energy we expend, the more food energy we consume. Therefore, if food intake is maintained at a constant level and exercise increases, that weight will be lost. It is as simple as that.

Further evidence as discussed in this chapter will also make it very clear why exercise at any level is an extremely valuable component of any weight maintenance program. So don't be discouraged from embarking on an exercise program because someone told you that you would have to become a triathlete to burn off the potato chip you ate last night.

The second myth is that exercise need not be strenuous. Leave it to our lazy human nature. Leisure creates our excess fat, then we shop around for a marketeer who will tell us that leisure can also remove it. Go to any health spa and you will see some members all dressed up in fancy leotards looking every bit the part of a potential huffing and puffing and sweating enthusiast. Instead, they leisurely

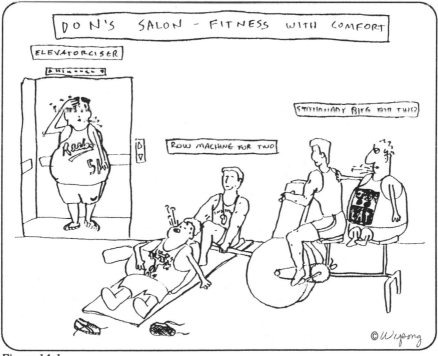

Figure 14-1

pull and push the various machines with weights small children could handle, never take a deep breath — much less create a drop of sweat — and dominate the machines that are designed with seats and reclining benches. There are now even "exercise" salons with "passive" machines that move your body parts for you.

No folks, although you don't have to be a marathoner, leisurely exercise is not the answer either. It takes slow, steady, incremental advances in numbers of repetitions, weights used, distance traveled, and compressed workout times to stimulate the body to new calorie burning metabolic baselines, increase lean muscle tissue, truly advance fitness, and dramatically improve your chances of obtaining and maintaining a healthy body.

Standard charts describing calorie consumption during workouts do not address peaks in exercise if a person is rigorously exercising. These peaks can amount to 1500 calories in an hour. A cross-country skier, for example, can expend up to 5,000 calories in a three-hour workout. Such calorie expenditure during vigorous athletic exercise can result in burning more calories than are normally consumed in three days.[1]

Continued vigorous exercise can also change the way food fuels are used. While a sedentary person normally converts fats consumed to fats deposited, a person who regularly engages in vigorous exercise increases the direct use of fatty acids consumed for fueling activity.[2]

Exercise sends a message to the body that it must prepare for activity rather than hibernation

Regular exercise sends a message to the body that it is, so to speak, an active, productive, alive body, and it needs to maintain a higher rate of metabolism for support. Inactivity, on the other hand, sends a message that the body is, in effect, hibernating, and it is time to conserve fuel stores and lower metabolic rate.

This is exactly how hogs and cattle are fattened. They're kept inactive in pens and feedlots.

From a psychological standpoint, exercise can get people thinking more about their body, how it looks, and how it feels. It makes

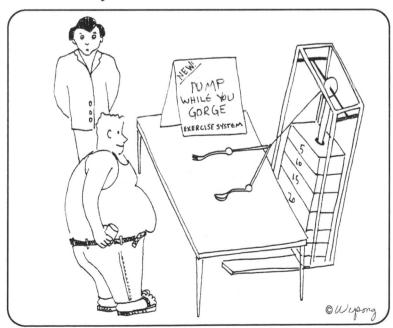

Figure 14-2

us start looking in mirrors, evaluating progress, and attempting to achieve goals. All this can result, if not carried to narcissistic extremes, in forward progress and great health benefits.

Regular exercise results in maintaining, if not building, the lean body muscular and bony mass. Although exercise may increase muscle size somewhat and give the appearance on a scale that change is not occurring, such muscle tone is both attractive and desirable to help maintain proper weight. If you just sit around and diet, 30 percent of the lost weight is muscle. You change from fat, muscle, and bone, to fat and bone. Not an attractive nor desirable change.

A lean, muscular body burns more energy at rest than an obese one

Lean body mass requires more energy from metabolism to maintain it, and thus more food fuel is burned even at rest. In effect, the internal thermostat is set higher. Up to 15 percent more calories are burned at rest after exercise. Muscle burns calories at rest; fat just sits there. Also, the larger the muscle, the more calories burned.

Whether it is productive work, play, or designed fitness regimens, exercise replaces the activity that would occur in the wild, whereby organisms are required to exercise to find shelter and food. To have shelter and food, without performing exercise to do it, is another genetic anachronism. We are not designed to have one without the other, but we do — and obesity is a result.

Exercise helps balance the parasympathetic with the sympathetic systems discussed previously. Exercise can result in its own neurochemical high, which helps replace some of the stimulation from eating and relaxation. We can actually get hooked on exercise.

There is a seemingly apparent exception to the relationship between food intake, exercise, and weight. It is confusing that with age there can be an inverse relationship between food intake and obesity. Older people often eat less but add more fat. But what is not taken into consideration is that as age increases, basal metabolic rate decreases and exercise levels decline. Thus as age progresses, eating less food can result in weight gain.

Hyperplastic (increased cell number) adipose tissue may be highly resistant to removal with exercise. These adipose cells are more close to their normal set-point size and thus are more resistant to change. In contrast, hypertrophic (increased size) fat cells are abnormally bloated with fat and more easily reduced. Unfortunately, hyperplastic adipose tissue is held in aesthestically unpleasing areas, and can be very discouraging to those attempting to remodel their bodies.[3] Nevertheless, a continuing and challenging exercise program (aerobic plus weight bearing is best), balanced with quality nutrition, will, over time, result in reshaping, and certainly will create significantly better results than simply dieting.

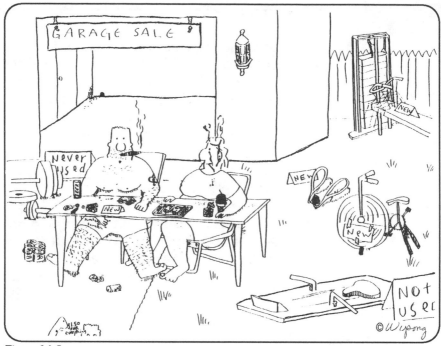

Figure 14-3

Although it is commonly believed that exercise will decrease appetite, it is unlikely that this is true except for a period immediately after intense exercise. Vigorous exercise actually will increase food intake, as would be expected. If this were not so, it would be possible to expend more energy than is consumed.[4] Moderate exercise in the obese will not necessarily increase appetite. Thus, it is possible to create a negative energy balance to a certain point that will help deplete excessive fat stores.

Intense exercise increases appetite

Exercise is, however, not a panacea for weight problems. It must be balanced against appropriate eating patterns. It can be carried to the extreme, becoming an endorphin high all on its own, without being balanced against appropriate nutrient intake. Eating disorders, such as anorexia and bulimia, can be consequences.

Exercise cannot replace thinking about what is eaten

On the other hand, exercise does not justify overconsumption. Though I don't like to get into the mathematics of calories, consider that during the same 30-minute period, an individual on a treadmill walking at four miles per hour will burn 210 calories; sitting in a chair doing nothing, he burns 39 calories. Thus there is only a net utilization of 171 calories. It takes considerable effort to burn off excessive consumption, particularly of fat calories. One ounce of fat holds 256 calories of energy. That makes for a lot of treadmill walking. It is much more reasonable to try not to create the fat stores, and to balance consumption with appropriate regular (lifelong) and reasonably vigorous exercise.[5]

Exercise out of balance can be as detrimental as no exercise

The health and body weight benefits of exercise are legion. What you gain from a regular exercise program may not be known — how can you know you have prevented that which may not occur — but the consequences of sedentary living are apparent and abound in our chronic degenerative disease-ridden society. Most people are concerned about embarking on an exercise program before having a check up. Perhaps a better approach is to have a check up if you decide not to exercise, to see if your body can survive it!

Caloric content of food can easily outdistance energy expenditure

Join a health club. Begin an outdoor sport such as walking, hiking, biking, cross country skiing, softball, soccer . . . anything. Then read and learn how to train to get better at it. Win a trophy. Power lift or body build (you will not get "muscle bound"). Join an aerobic or Jazzercise class. Get on a volleyball team. Play the most fitness-enhancing, underrated, undiscovered sport in America — competitive badminton.[6] Join a local club or call 1-800-621-2473 to find out how to begin.

Sure, by taking up an active sport you may get sore or injured once in a while. Big deal. All athletes contend with that. Better to deal with tennis elbow or a sprained ankle than a chest ripped open for bypass surgery or a life hooked up to an oxygen tank.

Do it. Do something to get started today. The social, psychological, and physical benefits add whole new dimensions and meaning to life.

1. Hatfield, Frederick C., Ph.D. *Ultimate Sports Nutrition.* Chicago: Contemporary Books, Inc., 1987.
2. Layzer, Robert B., M.D. "How Muscles Use Fuel." The New England Journal of Medicine 324 (1991): 411.
3. Bjorntorp, P. "Interrelation of physical activity and nutrition on obesity." Diet and Exercise: Synergism in Health Maintenance. American Medical Association (1982): 91-98.
4. Woo, R., et al. "Effect of exercise on spontaneous calorie intake in obesity." The American Journal of Clinical Nutrition (1982) 36: 470-477.
4a. Woo, R. et al. "Voluntary food intake during prolonged exercise in obese women." The American Journal of Clinical Nutrition (1982) 36: 478-484.
5. Pi-Sunyer, F. Xavier. "Obesity" in *Modern Nutrition in Health and Disease.* Philadelphia: Lea & Febiger, 1988, p. 809.
6. Wysong, R.L. *Wysong Review.* Midland, MI: The Wysong Institute, Nov. 1992.

15 - FIBER

The bandits who stole fiber are now praised for its return

The discovery of the benefits of fiber verifies the superior value of whole, natural foods

The current popularity of fiber as a healthy ingredient in foods is a verification of the value of whole, natural, raw foods. Modern food processing is guilty of fractionating natural, whole foods into components and selling them as isolated ingredients, or as new food combinations. The net result has been a decrease in dietary fiber. This decrease has now been linked to a wide range of degenerative diseases, including gastrointestinal disturbances, cancer, cardiovascular disease, and altered lipid metabolism.

It is interesting how modern technology/science/medicine now takes credit for the discovery of the health benefits of fiber. They credit their years of clinical controlled retrospective and prospective studies, metanalyses, and microbiological, physiological, and biochemical elucidations.

But look at what really has occurred. First, fiber is stripped out of foods and the "safety" of the new foods created is advocated to the masses. Then, after enough people have had their cancerous bowels removed, fiber is replaced back into the diet and cancer and other diseases related to constipation decrease. Who takes the credit? The processors and nutritionists, the very bandits who stole the fiber in the first place.

Rightful credit for the health benefits of fiber should go to the inherent wholesomeness that has always been within the perfect

111

composition of natural foods. We are now learning how well natural foods are constructed by paying the consequences of deviating too far from them. This is, in fact, a verification of the synorgonic theme of this book.

Supplemental fiber has potential dangers, as does fiber's absence

Although re-introducing whole foods, with their inherent natural fiber, is a wise nutritional step, it is controversial as to whether adding even higher levels of isolated fiber will benefit obesity. Theoretically, it would seem that if fiber, through its bulk and water-holding capacity, could create a lingering sense of satiety and increase the release of the appetite suppressing hormone cholecystokinin, that decreased food consumption should be the result. It would also theoretically seem that a fiber supplement could, by its bulk and its adsorbing characteristics, decrease the uptake of calorie-rich

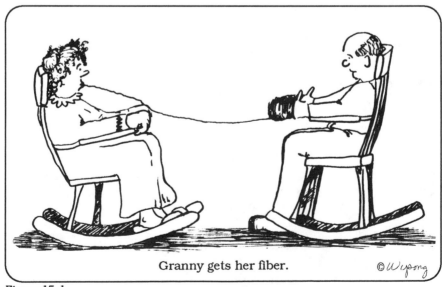

Granny gets her fiber.

Figure 15-1

nutrients. However, both of these assumptions are disputed. Some evidence indicates that isolated fiber neither decreases the absorption of calories nor decreases food intake.[1,2]

The value of high supplemental fiber in reducing diets is doubtful

High supplemental levels of dietary fiber bring potential health problems, as does any modeling of the diet contrary to its natural synorgonic archetypal design. Excessive fiber can result in bowel obstruction, bind essential nutrients such as minerals by its contained phytic acid, and may replace high quality, nutrient-dense food materials, rather than substituting for empty calories as intended.

Fiber as an isolated nutrient should only be used for specific short-term therapeutic purposes or as a supplement to a fiber de-

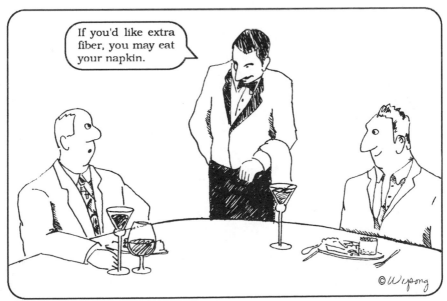

Figure 15-2

pleted diet. If taken, six to eight glasses of water should also be consumed daily to prevent potential obstructions.

The fiber inherent in whole foods is the correct healthful amount. Disease consequences from lack of fiber should not be taken as proof of fiber's merits, or as an opportunity to market yet another isolated nutrient, but as vindication of the value of whole, unaltered, natural foods and the wisdom of the Synorgon Diet.

---

1. Van Itallie, T.B. The American Journal of Clinical Nutrition 31 (1978): 543-552.
2. Van Itallie, T.B. The American Journal of Clinical Nutrition 32 (1979): 2723-2733.

16 - THE OBESE PERSONALITY

There are two conventional theories about what causes obesity. One is the "push" theory. It argues that people voluntarily push excess food into their bodies. The other is the "pull" theory. It explains obesity by the pull of metabolic disturbances that force us to overeat.

The push theory has traditionally been the most popular explanation — we overeat because we are weak and have no willpower. The pull theory is gaining ground, however, for many of the metabolic and physiological reasons addressed in the previous chapters.

In light of new discoveries linking obesity to organic problems, the push theory was a cruel explanation. It created societal contempt for huge numbers of individuals victimized by powerful organic obesity forces. Even professionals, biased by the push mentality, viewed the obese as not worthy of a sophisticated professional's time.

On the other hand, the pull theory creates the danger of the individual believing obesity is beyond his or her control – some people get struck by lightning, some by obesity.

But neither theory hits the mark. Both contain truth, but ignore the fundamental flaw of synorgonic imbalance.

Modern society permits excesses and imbalances unlike that which would be possible in the natural synorgonic setting. Taking advantage of conveniences and the opportunity to consume excesses of fractionated, isolated foods, sets the stage for altered metabolism and addiction (pull), and for overindulgence, weakness, laziness and dependence (push).

Understanding that obesity is a labyrinthine and puzzling disorder helps to avoid putting undue emphasis on any one cause. There are many causes, but synorgonic imbalance lies at the root of them all.

Overeating may begin with the conditioning to finish our plate

But let's look at how will and personality (push) do influence body weight.

Twisted eating logic can establish habits that are difficult to alter: We may overeat because of momentum; Once we've overstuffed ourselves, dessert doesn't matter; We may attack food like climbers do Mount Everest – Why eat what's left over? Because it's there; Or perhaps we devour every scrap to save starving children – "Clean your plate! Don't you know there are starving children in the world?"

Many obese individuals who have unsuccessfully dieted resign themselves to the belief that they are simply a victim of a metabolic (pull) disorder. Recent studies, however, have shown this is rarely the case.

Two hundred and twenty four obese individuals, some who had dieted 20 different times and supposedly restricted calories to 1,200 per day, were evaluated.

Participants in the study were followed by scientific assessment and then these results were compared to the diaries kept by the volunteers. The results showed that the true amounts of food and exercise were not registered in the diaries. It is important to note here that the amounts omitted from the diaries were not even registered in the subjects' consciousness.

This means that both underreporting of food consumed and overestimation of exercise are likely the causes of failure to succeed for most obese individuals attempting various low calorie diet programs. It is also important here to note, however, that this underreporting is not a conscious deception but is rather an "eye-mouth gap." Thus the conclusion cannot be reached that obese individuals are as such because of gluttony or sloth or a lack of character. This is true because even non-obese individuals underestimate caloric intake.

The "eye-mouth gap" is evidently an affliction that is particularly prevalent in the obese since underreporting by the obese is greater than underestimates by lean individuals, athletes and the elderly although these latter groups will also underreport. Women are also more likely to underestimate their intake than are men. But women are more likely to be obese by a five-to-one ratio compared to men.

Obese individuals who are convinced that their problem is something they must resign themselves to might do a more careful ap-

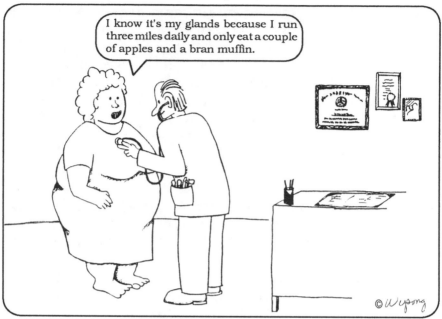

Figure 16-1

praisal of their eating patterns based upon this eye-mouth gap phenomenon. Even then, this is not to suggest that obesity is equally attainable in all individuals. For some individuals, there is a psychological predisposition, a susceptibility if you will, that results in the "eye-mouth gap."[1-3]

Social tensions can trigger eating disorders

Many obese people do not eat to combat hunger. They eat as a reaction to tension, anxiety, mental fatigue, and other modern stresses.[4] Although some people argue there is no classic "obesity personality"[5] and that behavioral modification is only mildly successful,[6] others argue that eating disorders have a strong social link, as evidenced by the fact that they do not occur in other areas of the world to the degree that they do in developed countries.[7] Even companion animals are believed more susceptible to obesity as a result of the boredom, conditioning, idleness, and nervousness present in modern-day households.[8]

Obesity is both psychological and biological

Much like smoking often begins in the early teen years when there is little understanding about long-term health consequences and an attitude of immortality is present, so too can eating excesses and disorders begin in the early years. In both situations, addiction can follow, and people and animals can become enslaved (pulled) to lifestyle patterns that began quite innocently or frivolously.

Balance must be achieved in childhood before obesity patterns become "normal"

A more balanced lifestyle shifted away from food-centered activities is a good start. As discussed in Chapter 11, neurotransmitter gratification can come from such activities as creative and challenging work, exercise, mutually caring relationships, games, and sports. Then, one is less likely to seek life's gratifications only through food. Food is meant to fuel enjoyable activity — not to be, in itself, life's most enjoyable activity.

A history of trial and failure, and fear of failure, can thwart progress before it even begins. Therefore, realistic expectations are important for any weight reduction or weight maintenance program. Strong chemical forces are at work to deter progress. An attitude of self-ownership, personal responsibility, self-control and self-efficacy is required. It means developing an expectation of success and a lifelong commitment to lifestyle modification.[9]

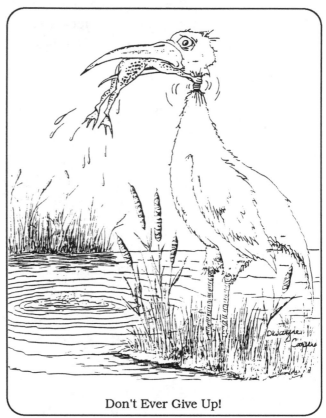

Don't Ever Give Up!

Figure 16-2

One cannot have an all-or-nothing attitude. Relapse should not mean that failure is inevitable and that a sound weight reduction or weight maintenance program should be abandoned. It is usual for self-esteem and one's determined psychological attitude to diminish each time weight is regained. Understanding in the beginning that these forces will be at work will prepare one for the inevitable ups and downs that will occur on the road to success.

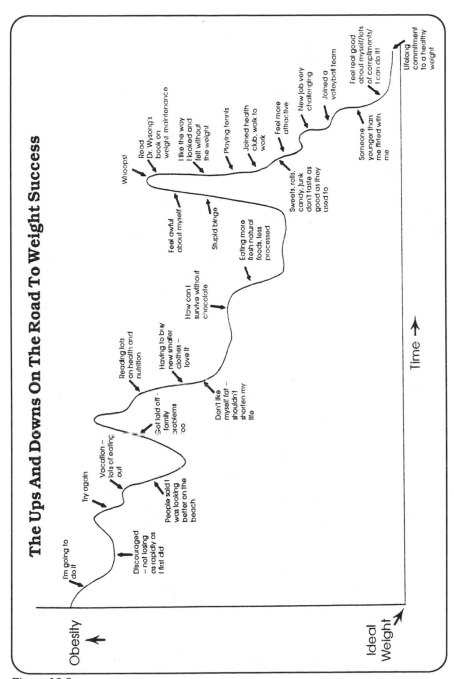

The Ups And Downs On The Road To Weight Success

Obesity ←

I'm going to do it

Try again

Discouraged -- not losing as rapidly as I first did

Vacation -- lots of eating out

People said I was looking better on the beach

Reading lots on health and nutrition

Got laid off -- family problems too

Having to buy new smaller clothes -- love it

Don't like myself fat -- shouldn't shorten my life

How can I survive without chocolate

Feel awful about myself

Stupid binge

Eating more fresh natural foods, less processed

Whoops!

Read Dr. Wysong's book on weight maintenance

I like the way I looked and felt without the weight

Playing tennis

Joined health club, walk to work

Feel more attractive

Sweets, rolls, candy, junk don't taste as good as they used to

New job very challenging

Joined a volleyball team

Feel real good about myself/lots of compliments/ I can do it!

Someone younger than me flirted with me

Lifelong commitment to a healthy weight

Time →

Ideal Weight ↗

Figure 16-3

Success is not a straight line from failure to perfection, but a series of hills and valleys on a more slow ascent to better health. Over time, an average of one percent weight loss per week in a committed program is a realistic expectation. It permits the necessary adaptations to occur in the new body that is created with each pound lost. Significant adjustments are required in metabolism and physiological functions in a body that may change to a fraction of its weight over a period of six months or a year.[10] This is one reason crash fad diets don't work. Metabolic and behavioral disturbances from rapid loss and imbalances can result in depression, intolerance to cold, and continual cravings and hunger.[11] Losing weight is not fun and it can even be likened to the pain of addictive drug withdrawal.

All worthwhile goals have their ups and downs

Changes take time before the new body becomes normal. That is, the body must see its new weight — rather than the obese weight — as the homeostatic (normal) baseline. In the meantime, powerful urges and cravings may exert pressure to return to the previously "normal" obesity homeostatic baseline. Thus, time, patience, commitment, and adjustments become essential to long-term success.

Time and patience are critical for the body to adapt to normal weight

Though powerful organic forces may cause us to resist weight loss, healthy weight can be achieved. As a disease, obesity has a cure rate of zero.[12] It can be controlled, however. Success requires a desire to change and a realization that we are all victims of synorgonic imbalance. More effort will be required and perhaps more discomfort felt by those who are more vulnerable than others.

By understanding the root cause of obesity — synorgonic imbalance — an initial gigantic stride is made toward recovery. Realizing that we are not simply hapless victims struck with a disorder opens the door for control. Resolve and commitment, combined with the patience required for metabolic readjustment, spell long-term success.

Beyond simply a new body, an added bonus of success is an empowered new you with the ability and confidence to better control your own health and life destiny. Achieving healthy weight, if done within the synorgonic perspective, is an opportunity to add a significant new dimension to your life.

---

1. Lightman, Steven W. "Discrepancy between self-reported and actual caloric intake and exercise in obese subjects." The New England Journal of Medicine 327 (1992): 1983-1989.
2. Danforth, Elliot, Jr. and Sims, Ethan, A.H. "Obesity and efforts to lose weight." The New England Journal of Medicine 327 (1992): 1947-1948.
3. Wysong, R.L. "The Eye-Mouth Gap" in the *Wysong Review*. Midland: Wysong Institute, March, 1993.
4. Bronell, K. and Foreyt, J. *Handbook of Eating Disorders*. New York: Basic Books, 1986, p. 376.
5. Pi-Sunyer, F. Xavier. "Obesity" in *Modern Nutrition in Health and Disease*. Philadelphia: Lea & Febiger, 1988.
6. Jeffrey, R.W., et al. Behav. Res. Ther. 16 (1978): 363-370.
7. Brumberg, J. "Fasting girls: reflections on writing the history of anorexia nervosa." Monographs of the Society for Research in Child Development 50 (1986): 93-104.
8. MacEwen, Gregory, VMD. "Fat cats and dogs." Petfood Industry 31 (1989): 28.

9. Mitchell, D., and Stuart, R.B. "Effect of self-efficacy on dropout from obesity treatment." Journal of Consulting and Clinical Psychology 52 (1984): 1100-1101.

10. Bjorntorp, P. "Interrelation of physical activity and nutrition on obesity" in *Diet and Exercise: Synergism in Health Maintenance.* Chicago: American Medical Association, 1982, pp. 91-98.

11. Greenwood, M.R.C., et al. "Weight control: A complex, various, and controversial problem" in *Obesity and Weight Control: The Health Professional's Guide to Understanding and Treatment.* Rockville, Maryland: Aspen Publisher, 1988, p. 5.

12. Frank, Arthur, M.D. "Futility and Avoidance." The Journal of the American Medical Association 269 (1993): 2132-2133.

17 - GAIN AND LOSS

95 percent of those who lose weight gain it back within one to five years

Twenty two pounds is the average practical limit of loss by dieting alone

Once excess weight is accumulated and then lost, maintaining the new weight for a period greater than five years is more difficult than curing many forms of cancer.[1,2]

Not understanding the powerful and complex forces behind obesity, combined with the quick fix mentality of our modern day, sets the stage for failure by individuals attempting to maintain normal body weight.

Ninety-five percent of those who lose excess weight have been found to gain it back within one to five years.[3] Unrealistic expectations (see Fig. 16-3), lack of commitment to fundamental lifestyle alterations, belief that obesity is a personality problem only, not a biochemical one, and of course, a lack of understanding of synorgonic imbalance can lead to a lifetime of dieting fads. Most diets do not address fundamental causes and thus, inevitably, result in the regain of the weight lost.

The yo-yo cycles of weight loss and regain are even more harmful to health than static obesity.[4] Both morbidity (disease) and early mortality increase with weight cycling.[5,6]

Each cycle of weight loss also decreases lean muscle body mass. If 20 pounds are lost, 13 pounds of that is fat and seven are water and muscle. When the 20 pounds are regained, 17 is fat and three are water and muscle. Not a good trade.

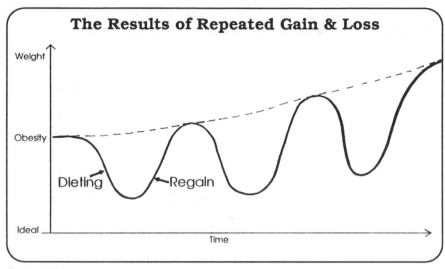

Figure 17-1

Dieting increases the efficiency of food utilization and storage

With each round, body fat increases and metabolic caloric needs fall.[7] Fat tissue requires few calories to maintain it, while muscle tissue demands higher calories even at rest. Even the thermogenic calorie burning response (see Chapter 9) is increased in the lean.[8]

If three percent of weight is lost, approximately six percent of our resting metabolic rate is also lost. With such compensation, the average practical limit of weight that can be lost by dieting alone (without increased exercise) is approximately 22 pounds.[9]

Fasting sends the body a signal that starvation is at hand. The body reacts by increasing the efficiency with which it uses food supplies, increases its energy storing capabilities, and decreases its resting metabolic rate so calories are not unnecessarily burned.[10] Then, when the diet is broken and food is eaten at the same level it was eaten before the diet began, more weight will be gained. The body remembers the threat of starvation and attempts to build reserves for the next round of starvation.[11]

After the diet is broken, the appetite for high-fat foods — recognized by the body as highly valuable if expecting starvation — actually increases.[12] Lipoprotein lipase activity also increases (see Appendix III), which increases the body's ability to store fat. Thus, weight loss during the next dieting cycle becomes much more difficult.

It is better not to diet than to diet and regain

The increase in food efficiency can be quite dramatic. In studies of rats, it has been found that there can be a fourfold increase in the efficiency of food utilization after repeated weight loss cycles.[13] Humans starving themselves as conscientious objectors increased body weight by an average of five percent after they broke the fast.[14]

The end result of yo-yo dieting is an increased percentage of body fat[15] and an increase in the waist-to-hip ratio (a big belly), which signals a foreboding increased risk of a variety of diseases.[16] (Review Chapter 6.)

Yo-yo cycling can also result from the very nature of weight loss itself. Initial loss is always very rapid and encouraging. Unfortunately, 70 percent of the initial loss is water.

Glycogen, a carbohydrate stored in muscle, is the first to be depleted. With each gram of glycogen lost, three to four grams of water are also lost. Then, a couple of weeks later, fat begins to be oxidized for energy needs. But fat, as you will recall from Chapter 9, is about three times more energy dense than glycogen, and thus only slowly diminishes.

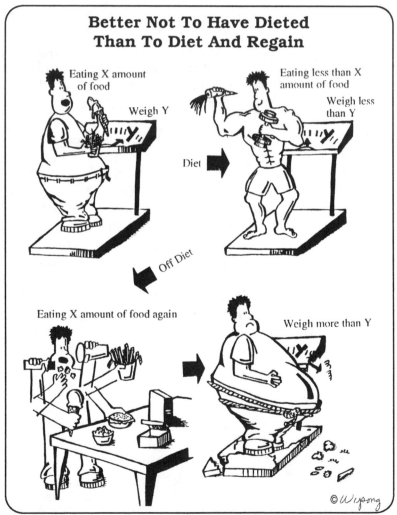

Figure 17-2

This is discouraging if there is not an understanding of what is to be expected. The diet may then be discontinued ("What's the use?") and restarted again another time, prompted by the memory of the early rapid success (which was actually only glycogen and water loss) of the previous diet.

The high recidivism rate for dieters does not mean losing weight is next to impossible. It speaks to a fundamental flaw in our society. We are literally surrounded by the reasons for obesity. Our world has become synorgonically imbalanced, making escape to normalcy very difficult — particularly if this flaw is not understood.

Any program to establish normal weight should therefore be well planned, thought through, and focused more on life-long synorgonic lifestyle modification than on any single food component, diet fad, or dramatic exercise program. Realistic goals and a life-time commitment are necessary not only to curtail the possible health consequences of obesity, but to prevent the increased risks which will result when more weight is gained as a consequence of dieting and gaining cycles.

---

1. Brownell, K.D. "The psychology and physiology of obesity: Implications for screening and treatment." Journal of The American Dietetic Association 84 (1984): 406-414.
2. Brownell, K.D. "Obesity: Understanding and treating a serious, prevalent, and refractory disorder." Journal of Consulting and Clinical Psychology 50 (1982): 820-840.

3. Benum, Sara. "Feast or Famine - An Examination of Weight Management Issues." Complementary Medicine 2 (January/February 1987): 14.

4. Brownell, K.D. "The psychology and physiology of obesity: Implications for screening and treatment." Journal of The American Dietetic Association 84 (1984): 406-414.

5. Lissner, Lauren, Ph.D. "Variability of body weight and health outcomes in the Framingham population." The New England Journal of Medicine 324 (1991): 1839.

6. Lee, I-Min, Sc.D. and Paffenbarger, Ralph S. Jr., M.D. "Change in body weight and longevity." The Journal of The American Medical Association 268 (1992): 2045.

7. Turner, Lori Waite, M.S., R.D. "Very-Low-Calorie Diets." Nutrition Clinics 4, No. 1 (January/February 1989): 7.

8. Maffeis, Cladio, et al. "Meal-induced thermogenesis in lean and obese prepubertal children." The American Journal of Clinical Nutrition 57 (1993): 481.

9. Donahoe, C.P., et al. "Metabolic consequences of dieting and exercise in the treatment of obesity." Journal of Consulting and Clinical Psychology 52, (1984): 834-835.

9a. Bray, G.A. "Future research in obesity" in Bray et al. 238-39.

10. Brownell, K.D, et al. "The Effects of Repeated Cycles of Weight Loss and Regain in Rats." Physiology & Behavior 38 (1986): 459-64.

11. Benum, Sara. "Yo-Yo Dieting — You Too Might Have an Eating Disorder." Medical Nutrition 5 (Winter 1990): 16.

11a. van Dale, Djoeke, et al. "Repetitive weight loss and weight regain: Effects on weight reduction, resting metabolic rate, and lipolytic activity before and after exercise and/or diet treatment." The American Journal of Clinical Nutrition 49 (1989): 409.

12. Reed, D.L., et al. "Weight Cycling in Female Rats Increases Dietary Fat Selection and Adiposity." Physiology and Behavior, 1988, Volume 42, pp. 389-395.

13. Brownell, Kelly, et al. "The effects of repeated cycles of weight loss and regain in rats." Physiology and Behavior 38 (1986): 459-464.

14. Callaway, C.W. "Biological adaptations to starvation and semistarvation" in Obesity and Weight Control: The Health Professional's Guide to Understanding and Treatment. Rockville, MD: Aspen Publishers, 1988, p. 105.

15. Benum, Sara. "Yo-Yo Dieting — You Too Might Have an Eating Disorder." Medical Nutrition 5 (Winter 1990): 14.

16. Rodin. J. et al. "Weight Cycling and Fat Distribution." International Journal of Obesity 14 (April 1990): 303-310.

The immune system is designed to distinguish between self and nonself. This is as essential as a soldier understanding who is on his side, and who is the enemy. If the immune system works in this way — protecting self and destroying nonself — everything is fine. However, a range of autoimmune (immune to self) diseases has been recognized in the last few decades and their incidence is increasing. The immune system in these diseases turns against the body and attacks tissues, resulting in disease. Such diseases include forms of arthritis, multiple sclerosis, myasthenia gravis, lupus erythematosus, diabeties mellitus...and secondarily even obesity.

The immune system is affected by a wide range of subtleties

The immune system is comprised of cells and biochemicals designed to attack potential body invaders. It was once thought to be outside the control of other organs. This is no longer believed to be the case, however. The immune system is now known to be intimately linked with many other systems, including the endrocrine and neurological systems.

Interrelatedness is a fundamental of our synorgonic natural world. Nothing is truly isolated. Everything is intricately related and balanced in such a way, at least in the natural context, to help preserve health. It is little wonder, then, that new discoveries show that how we think and eat, and even magnetic fields and length of daylight, can affect the immune system's ability to combat disease.

Could autoimmunity be related to our modern setting? Clues may be found in the continuing daily assault of a wide range of chemical toxins in our food, water, and air, and compromised levels of nutrients responsible for maintaining a healthy immune system. Perhaps the immune system becomes confused by various inoculations wherein foreign genetic material is actually introduced into the genome making "self" cells really not "self." Some believe vaccinations may be at the root of certain immune system self-destructive attacks.[1,2]

As the environment degrades, stress to the immune system increases

Auto-antibodies (antibodies against our own tissue) have now been identified which act against indigenious weight regulatory sites such as the thyroid gland.[3] Thyroid hormones are part of the metabolic regulatory mechanism. When thyroid hormones decrease as a result of autoimmune destruction of thyroid tissue, metabolism decreases and food fuels burn less efficiently. Fat is thus more readily deposited.

Auto-immune alteration of weight regulatory mechanisms may lie at the root of many weight control problems

Diabetes, obesity and autoimmunity are also linked. The beta cells in the pancreas responsible for producing insulin, and receptors on cells in body tissues responsible for receiving insulin, can be self-attacked through autoimmunity.[4] Obesity can result from either.[5] The loss of insulin-producing beta cells in the pancreas as a cause of diabetes is well known. No beta cells means no insulin which means diabetes. Tissue loss of insulin receptors is less well known. With decreased insulin receptors, the pancreas is stimulated to produce more and more insulin until it is exhausted and unable to produce sufficient amounts. The end result is diabetes.[6]

Diabetes leads to obesity because insulin also affects the metabolism and uptake of amino acids into cells. With insulin depletion and tissue resistance to it, amino acids elevate in the blood decreasing the ratio of tryptophan in relation to others. Insulin increases the movement of non-tryptophan amino acids into tissues more rapidly than tryptophan, thus increasing the relative tryptophan levels in blood.

Mood swings due to varying levels of glucose and serotonin create cycles of eating binges

This decreased tryptophan ratio makes it more difficult for tryptophan to pass the blood-brain barrier and to produce serotonin. Lower levels of serotonin create depression as discussed in Chapter 12. This can signal increased eating of carbohydrate, which the body believes will increase the secretion of insulin. Insulin would decrease the level of other amino acids in relation to tryptophan so that more serotonin could be produced and mood lifted. But this cannot happen with insulin resistance. Thus, eating is continually stimulated and weight is gained.[7]

Mood swings are also exacerbated by the brain's glut for glucose. The brain accounts for some 60 percent of the utilization of glucose used by the entire body in the resting state. As blood sugar levels swing wildly due to refined carbohydrates in the

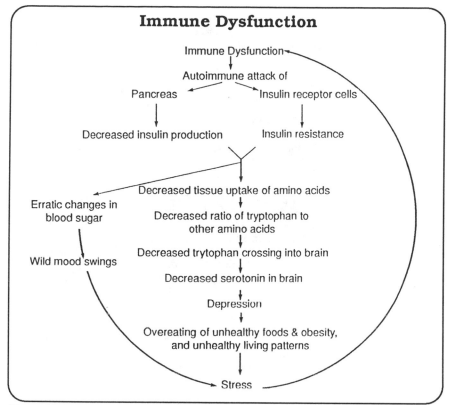

Immune Dysfunction

Immune Dysfunction

↓

Autoimmune attack of

Pancreas ← → Insulin receptor cells

↓ ↓

Decreased insulin production   Insulin resistance

Decreased tissue uptake of amino acids

↓

Erratic changes in blood sugar   Decreased ratio of tryptophan to other amino acids

↓

Decreased trytophan crossing into brain

↓

Wild mood swings   Decreased serotonin in brain

↓

Depression

↓

Overeating of unhealthy foods & obesity, and unhealthy living patterns

↓

→ Stress

Figure 18-1

Obesity, diabetes, thyroid function and auto-immunity are probably all interlinked

diet and insulin abnormalcy, one would expect that moods could be affected, contributing to abberant eating behavior.

Thus obesity, diabetes, thyroid dysfunction, and autoimmunity are all part of the same disease complex. Successful weight management in such cases may ultimately hinge upon restoring the immune system to proper function. This is a complex problem obviously not resolved by such popular approaches as eating high-fiber muffins or drinking a high-protein milkshake.

The fundamental synorgonic imbalance must be addressed and corrected to achieve a lasting solution.

---

1. The Humanitarian Publishing Company, R.D. #3, Quakertown, PA 18951.
2. Vaccine Research Institute, Josephine Szczesney, P. O. Box 4182, Northbrook, IL 60065.
3. Benker, G., et al. "Response of Total and "free" thyroid hormones and diodotyrosine to bovine TSH in subclinical hypothyroidism." ACTA Endocrinoligica 112 (1986): 509.
4. Darnall, Lyn. "New Horizons in the treatment of obesity." Complementary Medicine 2 (1987): 42.
5. Lundgren, Hans, et al. "Dietary habits and incidence of non-insulin-dependent diabetes mellitus in a population study of women in Gothenburg, Sweden." The American Journal of Clinical Nutrition 49 (1989): 708.
6. Pi-Sunyer, F. Xavier. "Obesity" in *Modern Nutrition in Health and Disease.* Philadelphia: Lea & Febiger, 1988, pp. 801-802.
7. Anderson, G. Harvey. "Metabolic Regulation of Food Intake" in *Modern Nutrition in Health and Disease.* Philadelphia: Lea & Febiger, 1988, pp. 565-566.

One in four youths is overweight

The weight patterns of children often follow those of the adults in the home. It is estimated that more than 11 million children in the U.S. between the ages of six and 17 are overweight. That is one in every four youths. Between 1963 and 1980, obesity in 6-to-11-year-olds increased 54 percent and super-obesity increased 100 percent.[1] In one study of fourth grade girls, it was found that 70 percent of them worried about their weight, and 80 percent of girls dieted by the time they were 18. Eighty percent of obese young children will end up being obese adults.[2,3]

Fat children make fat adults

Considering the health ramifications of excess weight, its control becomes a serious responsibility for parents. If it is not addressed during youth, living patterns and physiological adaptions can occur which make it extremely difficult to readjust weight with each passing year that excess weight is maintained.[4]

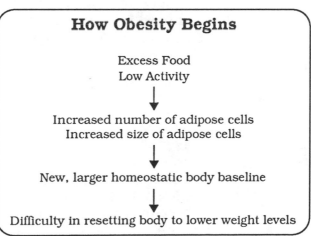

How Obesity Begins

Excess Food
Low Activity

↓

Increased number of adipose cells
Increased size of adipose cells

↓

New, larger homeostatic body baseline

↓

Difficulty in resetting body to lower weight levels

Figure 19-1

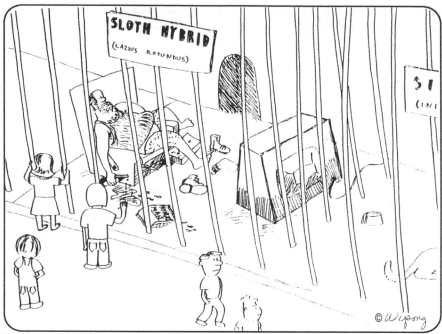

Figure 19-2

**Obesity
in the
young
can
cause
disease
decades
later**

Adipose tissue can not only fill to capacity, but these fat-storing cells can increase in number as discussed in Chapter 2. After they are adapted to obesity in a child, these tissues will metabolically be "comfortable" only with the obese state. The baseline is changed and can create lifelong pressure to maintain excess weight.

Additionally, very real damage can occur as a result of obesity in youth that may not manifest itself until adult or even middle-aged life. Permitting obesity in young children can be the direct cause of diabetes, a heart attack, or cancer. A cute, plump child we spoil with obesity-causing foods and a sedentary life is therefore really not so cute — it's deadly serious. Intelligent foresight and rearing with a view to the child's adult healthy future is one of the best gifts we can give children.[5]

The solution is appropriate balances — not magic dietary regimens. Adults must establish lifestyle patterns that encourage appropriate weight balance as a model for children to emulate. Making television viewing a central family activity, for example, can lead to obesity. Studies have shown that metabolic rate decreases, with fat deposition increasing, if snacks and meals are eaten in front of a TV.[6]

When synorgonic balance is achieved, weight control does not become an issue or an obsession for young minds, but it is the given, which it should be, when eating and living patterns reflect natural balances.

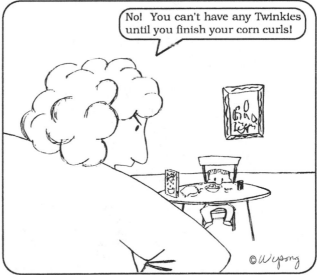

Figure 19-3

An important caveat must be noted. Attempting to limit children's fat intake has the potential of compromising important nutritional growth factors. Fat-soluble vitamins, such as A, D, E, and K; phospholipids; and essential fatty acids are particularly important in young growing bodies, and especially for neurological development.

Severe restriction of all fatty foods may benefit certain adults, but it could compromise the health of a youngster. Children must be permitted pretty much free choice and adequate availability of foods to ensure nutritional variety and nutrient sufficiency.

This will work without obesity consequences with a diet of choices from a variety of fresh, whole, natural foods. The modern processed fare of fractionated, embalmed, chemically-laden, fat-enriched food artifacts neither insures adequate nutrition nor prevents obesity, regardless of how the child's diet is manipulated.[7]

---

1. "Obesity among children: it's growing bigger." Tufts University Diet & Nutrition Letter, Vol. 5, No. 9 (1987): 7.
2. Mossberg, H. Acta Paediatr. Scand. (Suppl. II) 35 (1948): 1-122.
3. Abraham, S. and Nordsieck, M. Public Health Report 75 (1960): 263-273.
4. Mossberg, Hans-Olof. "40-Year Follow-up of Overweight Children." The Lancet 8661 (1989): 491.
5. Must, Aviva, Ph.D., et al. "Long-term Morbidity and Mortality of Overweight Adolescents." The New England Journal of Medicine 327 (1992): 1350.
6. Associated Press Wire Story, April 2, 1992.
7. Klesges, Robert C. "Parental influence on food selection in young children and its relationships to childhood obesity." The American Journal of Clinical Nutrition 53 (1991): 859.

20 - TOO MUCH OF TOO LITTLE

A potato contains more than 150 chemicals, not just starch

Processed, fractionated foods are fraught with risks of deficiencies and excesses — in other words, imbalance. Natural foods are balanced and complex in nature. Modern foods are imbalanced and simplified.

It is, for example, possible to extract the starch from potatoes and create an instant potato mix. But potatoes are more than the resulting starch. Whole potatoes contain more than 150 separate chemicals. This complex aggregate is the nutrition in the potato, not simply the powdered white fluff that can be boxed.

Another example: When bread is produced, more than 24 nutrients are lost and then two or three synthethic B vitamins and iron are replaced. The result is then called "fortified," as if it were even better than what was in the original grain. It's like tearing down rock walls surrounding a castle, replacing them with a picket fence, and calling the result fortified...an incredible abuse and intentional misuse of the English language.

More than 24 nutrients are lost when bread is produced

Whole natural food is like a complete alphabet. Although some letters can be removed and many words still formed, such removal can seriously impair language. Remove just the letter "U" and almost 3000 words are lost. Similarly, although life may function with many food components removed, the fullness of life, its optimal health, will be compromised by doing so.

Natural creatures — which we all are, of course — have adapted through eons to natural, raw, whole foods. We could not have a nutritional requirement beyond that which natural foods could provide. Otherwise, we would not exist today. But modern logic argues that we must eat from an arbitrary four food groups daily, and that fortified, fractionated, processed foods have merits equal to or beyond those of natural foods themselves.

Natural foods are self-processing

But natural foods are far more replete with nutritional value than modern processed, fractionated foods. They contain a spectrum of vitamins and minerals; active enzymes to assist in digestion; proteins; carbohydrates; essential fatty acids; and an array of accessory nutrients, most of which we do not yet fully understand. Natural food contains the nutritional machinery which is necessary for its digestion, assimilation, and utilization. But when we remove components of a natural food and feed only fractions, those nutritional benefits are lost.

Nutrient deficiency diseases are often linked directly to processing

Worldwide epidemics have been created by ignoring the wisdom inherent in the complexity of natural foods. For example, when whole rice is milled, more than 75 percent of its vitamin B_1 is lost. In Japan alone, more than 15,000 people per year died from this deficiency, known as beriberi, in the early to mid-1900's.

Scurvy from vitamin C depleted foods, pellagra from vitamin B_3 depleted foods, zinc deficiency, copper deficiency, iron deficiency, and so on are serious maladies that have afflicted humans and animals since the advent of the processed, fractionated diet.

Sugar, protein, carbohydrates, fats, vitamins, or minerals do not exist as isolated nutrients in nature. But they abound in the commercial marketplace both as readily available ingredients for processed foodstuffs, and as end-product consumer foods and supplements. In the U.S. alone, more than 20 pounds of candy are eaten per person, per year; more than $700 million a year are spent on croissants made basically from fractionated flour and processed oil; each person consumes approximately 120 pounds of sugar per year; we consume 500 12-ounce soft drinks per person each year; as a country we eat more than 75 acres of pizza every day made primarily of food fractions; and every man, woman, and child on the average consumes about 15 gallons of grease, tallow, lard, and hydrogenated oil yearly.

Individual nutrients do not exist as isolated entities in nature

The medical and nutritional community hammers away at the need for individuals to eat from the "four food groups" daily. But evidence is convincing that the "four food groups" have been strongly influenced by economic powers who benefit from having their products listed in these four food groups. These powers include the meat and dairy industries.

The naive public can consider its nutritional responsibilities covered by eating a cheeseburger with lettuce and tomatoes on it, since this contains the four food groups. But a steady diet of such burgers predisposes to an array of diseases, because it is micronutrient poor, low in fiber, high in fat, and contaminated with a variety of potential toxins derived from processing.

A hamburger with cheese and lettuce meets the popular "four food groups" nutritional criterion

There is ongoing controversy regarding the relative merits of natural foods as opposed to synthetic. The conventional medical and nutritional communities argue that a calorie is a calorie is a calorie, and a vitamin is a vitamin is a vitamin regardless of source. They argue that it makes little difference to the body, in terms of short or long term health, whether it consumes a food manufactured in a laboratory, or one picked from the vine. But scientific opinion often lags far behind current, scientific evidence. Such is the case with this issue.

Nutrients as they are complexed within foodstuffs are superior to isolated synthetics

Ample scientific evidence proves that natural foods have merits surpassing those in the test tubes of chemists.[1] (For sources, see page 258, nos. ED001 and ED057, and page 259, no. ED050.) Naturally complexed vitamin C, for example, has been found to be more effective than synthetic.[2] The benefits of broccoli in cancer prevention are by and large lost when broccoli is cooked. Cholesterol as a part of raw, natural foods is nutritious, but after it is oxidized in processing, it becomes toxic — leading to a variety of pathologies, including atherosclerosis. A deficiency in the amino acid taurine in cat foods causes eye, reproductive, and heart diseases.

This is the direct result of the effects of processing on natural foods.

Links being found between nutrition and health verify the value of natural foods

Richly colored fruits and vegetables contain more than 300 isomers of natural carotenoids. Synthetic forms contain one, a trans- form. The natural carotenoids contain cis- forms and are found to be more active against cancer than the synthetic ones.[3] Lecithin from natural sources is superior to synthetic choline. Fish oil in whole fish is more effective than extracted oils in capsules. Even subtleties are important in metabolism, including the subtle, tertiary, three-dimensional structure of proteins lost easily in processing.[4]

Food Sources and Processing Losses

Concentrated food sources of taurine include: beef muscle, lamb muscle, pork muscle, chicken muscle, oysters and clams. Below are the results of processing on various sources.

	Uncooked Mean*	Baked Mean*	Boiled Mean*
Pork Muscle	496	219	118
Oysters	698	264	89
Clams	2400	1017	446

(*mg/kg net weight)

Figure 20-1

Virtually every current recommendation demonstrating links between nutrition and health directly or indirectly argues the case for the value of natural foods. An excellent example is the current fiber craze. Fiber deficiency only exists because fiber has been processed out of the modern diet (see Chapter 15).

The supposed value of omega -3 fish oils in heart disease, allergies, and a broad range of other health problems was discovered as a direct result of fractionating foods and creating domestic food sources depleted of these fatty acids. For example, wild game meat may have as much as five times the amount of polyunsaturated fatty acids as domestic meat, and may contain as much as four or more percent omega -3 fatty acids. Domestic meat may contain zero.[5]

Comparison of Domestic and Wild Animal Meat

	% Protein	% Fat	% Polyunsaturated fatty acids as a % of total fat
Domestic Meat (Lamb, pork, beef)	16	27	7
Wild Game Meat (Cape buffalo, warthog, deer, grouse, horse, giraffe, etc.)	24	4	37

Figure 20-2

Greek range chickens eat grass, insects, figs, barley, corn, and the green leafy vegetable highest in omega -3 fatty acids — purslane. These chickens' eggs contain 17.87 milligrams per gram of omega -3 fatty acids. By comparison, an average American egg contains 1.74 milligrams per gram. The ratio of omega -6 to omega -3 is 1:3 in the Greek egg and 19:4 in the American egg. One hundred grams of Greek egg yolk contain

1,787 milligrams of omega -3 fatty acids, whereas one average commercial fish oil capsule which we may take to try to supplement contains 300 milligrams.

Cultured fish fed modern agricultural products suffer a decrease in the amount of omega -3 fatty acids — the fish oil factor — compared to their wild counterparts.[6]

Minimal nutrient intakes are not being met by a large segment of the population

The sodium-to-potassium ratio should be 10:1 for best health. It is now inverted with sodium excess common in the modern diet. Why does this happen? Look at corn. Fresh corn contains 280 milligrams of potassium and one milligram of sodium per 1,100 grams. Canned, it contains 97 milligrams of potassium and 235 milligrams of sodium. Flaked, it contains no potassium and 1,000 milligrams of sodium.

These disparities between products of the modern farm and wild, more natural foods, plus the changes that result in food from processing, make it clear how far the modern diet has veered from its original character.

Examination of the nutritional intake of populations on modern processed foods verifies widespread deficiencies and imbalances. One study of 20,000 individuals found that none received 100 percent of the minimal daily recommended allowance of 10 nutrients.[7] Another study found that 50 percent of the population consumed less than half the minimal recommended daily allowance of vitamin C.[8] And other studies have shown that the "normal" diet is usually low in vitamins B_1, B_2, B_6, and C.[9,10] More than 40 percent of the population take nutritional supplements with the intuitive suspicion that the modern, processed food fare is not adequate...and they're right.

We are a society of overconsumption and under-nutrition

Modern society creates an abundance of food. Whether this food is even actually food by definition or not, is another question. Much of it is nutrient depleted, imbalanced, and tainted with a variety of toxins from both the environment and as a result of the action of processing on the chemicals within the food itself. We can consume plenty of carbohydrates, protein, and fats, but these elements can be distorted from their natural character, and can be depleted of the micronutrients necessary to properly metabolize them — like choking an engine. We receive too much of too little. We are guilty of over consumption and under nutrition. We have created a new phenomenon: affluent malnutrition.

Fractionated, processed foods can directly contribute to difficulties in weight management. Some fractionated foods can be highly addictive, such as sugars and other refined carbohydrates, oils, and fats. We have discussed the effects of sugars on the brain, mood, and appetite chemicals. Research has also identified a brain protein, galanin, which is associated with people craving fatty foods.[11]

Obese individuals usually consume less than half the amount of micronutrient-rich

How We Have Changed Our Food Environment

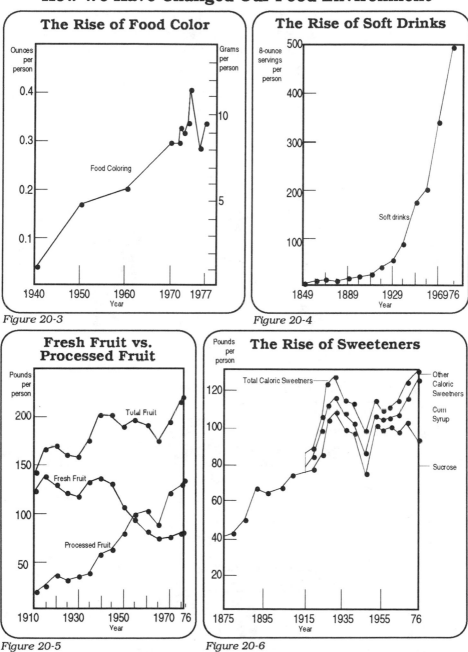

Figure 20-3

Figure 20-4

Figure 20-5

Figure 20-6

Graphs from *The Changing American Diet*, published by Center for Science in the Public Interest, Washington D. C. 1983

fruits and vegetables they should, but double the amount of refined carbohydrates and fats. As a result, they receive only about 25 percent of the minimal recommended requirement of several vitamins and minerals.[12]

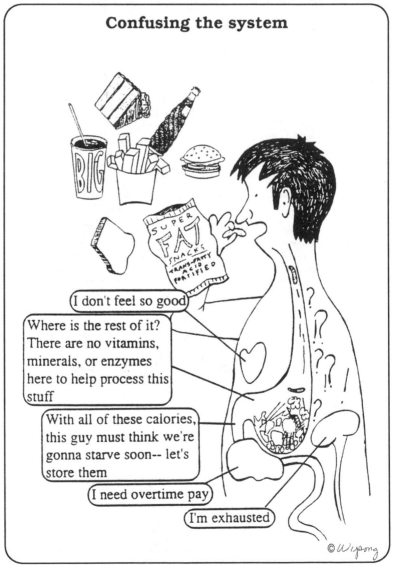

Figure 20-7

This problem is further complicated by low calorie (1,200 or less) diets. Such diets, researchers have shown, simply cannot meet the RDA's . . . and the RDA's are extremely conservative, even far too low according to the most current studies.[13]

There is also a suspicion that some who over-consume are unconsciously seeking nutrients for which they are deficient; they are trying to unchoke the engine. Micronutrient deficiency causes a hidden hunger.

But to relieve the hunger, the foods they usually turn to are chronically deficient. Thus they simply continue in their over-consumptive pattern which led to, and now maintains, obesity. Thus it is possible that although a person or animal may appear engorged with nutrients, his weight disorder may actually be a reaction to nutrient deficiency — not food excess.

High-quality, balanced nutrition, from foods as close to their natural character as possible, and vitamin-mineral-enzyme supplement products (designed from natural foods to the degree possible, not synthetics) thus become an important starting point in any weight management program. (For sources, see page 263, no. 4.)

---

1. The American Journal of Clinical Nutrition (May, 1971): 562.
2. Vinson, Joe A., Ph.D. and Bose, Pratima, Ph.D. "Comparative bioavailability to humans of ascorbic acid alone or in a citrus extract." The American Journal of Clinical Nutrition 48 (1988): 601.

3. Journal of Nutrition 120 (1990): 889.
4. Kossiakoff, A.A. "Tertiary Structure Is a Principal Determinant to Protein Deamidation." Science 240 (1988): 191.
5. The New England Journal of Medicine 312.5, p. 285.
6. van Vliet, Trinette and Katan, Martijn B. "Lower ratio of n-3 to n-6 fatty acids in cultured than in wild fish." The American Journal of Clinical Nutrition 51 (1990): 1.
7. Food Processing 48 (1987): 139.
8. Gey, K. Fred, M.D., et al. "Plasma levels of antioxidant vitamins in relation to ischemic heart disease and cancer." The American Journal of Clinical Nutrition 45S (1987): 1368-1377.
9. van der Beek, Eric J., M.D., et al. "Thiamin, riboflavin, and vitamins B_6 and C: impact of combined restricted intake on functional performance in man." The American Journal of Clinical Nutrition 48 (1988): 1451.
10. van Dokkum, W., et al. "Vitamin restriction and functional performance in man." The American Journal of Clinical Nutrition 49S (1989): 1138-1139.
11. Ezzel, C. "Craving fat? Blame it on a brain protein." Science News 142 (1992): 311.
12. Travers, K.D. Raine, et al. "Dietary Characteristics and Nutrient Intake of Morbidly Obese Patients." Journal of the Canadian Dietetic Association 48 (1987): 113-116.
13. Ibid.

21 - GOOD FATS, BAD FATS

What has been done to lipids prior to consumption is a key health question

Lipids come in many forms. In their form within natural foods they serve as fuel, as well as contribute to and improve health by providing proper substrates for metabolic functions and dynamic cellular structural components. But after fats and oils are baked, boiled, frozen, fried, freeze-dried, canned, solvent-extracted, extruded, deodorized, hydrogenated, and exposed to light and oxygen, we have another matter. The manipulation of natural lipids makes them no longer natural, but rather something new, synthetic, and foreign to biological experience (see Figure 21-1).

Lipids are not a luxury, nor are they innocuous. They are not a food component to avoid merely to prevent accumulation on bellies, bottoms or chins. Fat is not simply a repository of calories, forcing us to embark on weird reducing diets or to spend countless hours on a treadmill.

The lipid structure of all membranes directly reflects the diet

Lipids are complex and dynamic biochemicals found ubiquitously and necessarily throughout the body. Their caloric density is only one of their many important aspects. The composition of the cell membranes of all the 60 trillion cells throughout the body is a direct reflection of the kinds of lipids and associated nutrients we eat. The lipid-concentrated cell membranes, which govern the flow of all substances into and out of cells, are the very gatekeepers of life. The membranes of organelles within cells (such as mitochondria and lysosomes) are likewise composed of lipids. Lipids are essential to visual and neural functions. They are a part of glandular secretions, help muscles recover, retain moisture in the skin, and are necessary for growth, tissue repair and reproduction. Lipids serve as important substrates and modulators throughout the body; they touch, in one way or another, virtually every life process.

Lipids are vital in every life process

Lipids must therefore be thought of as far more than passive, unwanted components of food. They are vital nutrients every bit as necessary and dynamic as vitamins, minerals, and proteins.

Processing changes healthy natural lipids into something quite different

The most vital of lipids, the unsaturated essential fatty acids, for example, can undergo a variety of degradations rendering them non-nutritious at best and toxic at worst. The double bonds in essential fatty acids are highly fragile and particularly susceptible to heat, light, and oxygen-prevailing elements in food processing. (See Appendix I for further biochemical details on lipids.) Oxygen attacks the double bond-forming toxic free-radicals capable of widespread chain-reaction biochemical damage (see Figures 21-1 and 21-2).

To further aggravate the problem, oxidation is speeded by heat and accelerated a thousandfold by light. Those tasty french fries just pulled out of the boiling three-day-old fat vat aren't quite so tasty to our genetic material, immune system, visual neurons, and cell membranes (see Figure 21-3).

As a part of natural foods, essential fatty acids are protected both within the physical

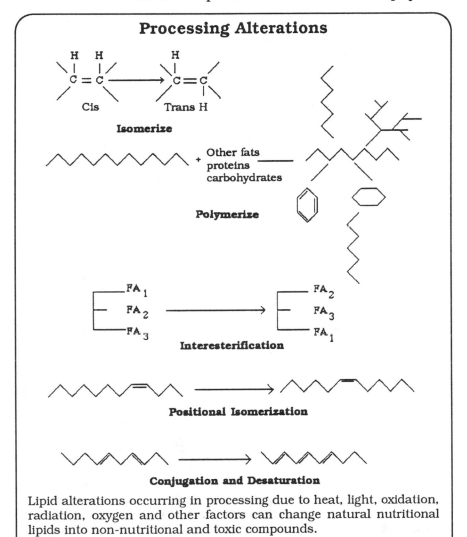

Processing Alterations

Isomerize

Polymerize

Interesterification

Positional Isomerization

Conjugation and Desaturation

Lipid alterations occurring in processing due to heat, light, oxidation, radiation, oxygen and other factors can change natural nutritional lipids into non-nutritional and toxic compounds.

From *Lipid Nutrition: Understanding fats and oils in health and disease* by Dr. Randy L. Wysong, Inquiry Press, 1990.

Figure 21-1

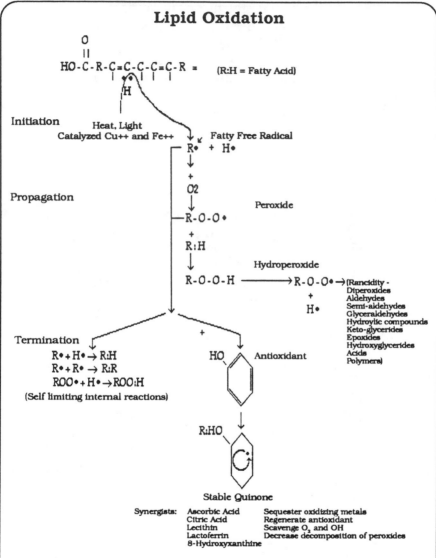

Lipid Oxidation

Unsaturated fatty acids readily undergo oxidative degradation in an accelerating cycle if not checked by antioxidant chemicals. Stabilization of commercial oils is as important as the body's need to stabilize its tissue lipids.

From *Lipid Nutrition: Understanding fats and oils in health and disease* by Dr. Randy L. Wysong, Inquiry Press, 1990.

Figure 21-2

matrix of the seed, nut, or leaf, and also
biochemically by natural antioxidants such
as vitamins C and E, beta carotene, and

Free Radical Damage To Membranes

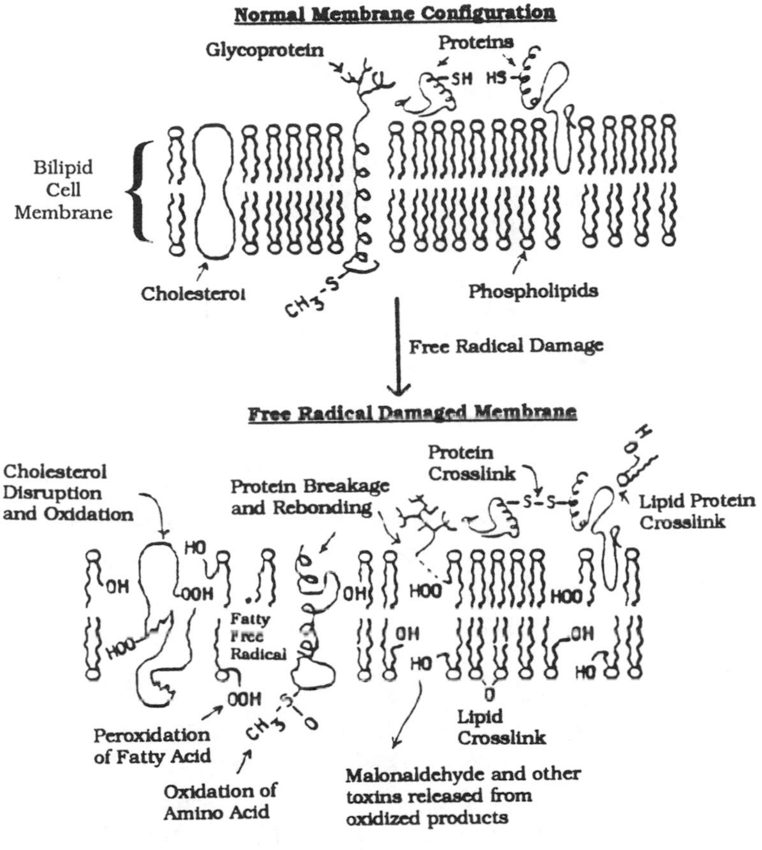

Tissue membranes are complex bilayer molecular structures capable of
undergoing disruption from free radicals. The resulting membrane loses
structural and functional integrity resulting in characteristic aging,
wrinkles, drying and predisposition to neoplasia. This schematic of what
happens to skin tissue due to free radical damage reflects what can
happen throughout body tissues. Compare to Figure I-10 in Appendix I.

From *Lipid Nutrition: Understanding fats and oils in health and disease* by Dr. Randy L. Wysong, Inquiry
Press, 1990.

Figure 21-3

The "no preservatives" food changes the frying pan to fire

certain enzymes, amino acids, and minerals. Processing removes, alters, or destroys food's natural protection, leaving the fragile molecules vulnerable to degradation. Synthetic antioxidants are used by processors to help protect lipid molecules, but these are increasingly being linked to their own set of dangers. Perhaps even worse is the "no preservatives" trend. Although this marketing fad may avoid the dangers of synthetic antioxidants, it leaves lipids free to degrade, which is perhaps an even greater health danger.

The significance of the foregoing to obesity lies in the dangers of carrying unnaturally altered and toxic free-radical-generating compounds in copious amounts within our body. Since the fats accumulated in the obese are predominantly those derived from processed diets, a fat body can be thought of as a processed body, complete with isomerized, polymerized, esterified, conjugated, desaturated and hydrogenated lipid riffraff.

Excess fat on the body is usually excess processed fat

When altered and oxidized lipids are incorporated into membranes and fat stores throughout the body, they have the potential for causing a variety of disease states. Such lipid toxins are probably the root cause of the various pathologies to which the obese are particularly susceptible, as discussed in Chapter 6.

A case in point is atherosclerosis. Although the popular notion linking cholesterol and saturated fats to this disease has cast suspicion on all forms of dietary fat,

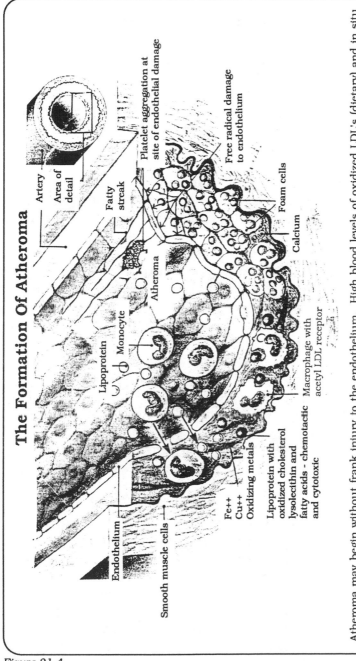

The Formation Of Atheroma

Artery

Area of detail

Endothelium

Smooth muscle cells

Fe++
Cu++
Oxidizing metals

Lipoprotein with
oxidized cholesterol
lysolecithin and
fatty acids - chemotactic
and cytotoxic

Macrophage with
acetyl LDL receptor

Lipoprotein

Monocyte

Atheroma

Calcium

Foam cells

Free radical damage
to endothelium

Fatty
streak

Platelet aggregation at
site of endothelial damage

Atheroma may begin without frank injury to the endothelium. High blood levels of oxidized LDL's (dietary) and in situ oxidation of LDL's in the vessel wall are scavenged by macrophages with specific receptors for oxidized LDL's (acetyl LDL receptors). Macrophages engorge with oxidized LDL's, form foam cells and create free radical damage to the overlying endothelium. Once this occurs, platelets aggregate, growth factors and arachidonic cascade products propagate damage leading to atheroma and eventual vessel closure. (Modified from Steinberg/Grey)

From *Lipid Nutrition: Understanding fats and oils in health and disease* by Dr. Randy L. Wysong, Inquiry Press, 1990.

Figure 21-4

consideration is not usually given to the form of these fats. A natural fat, such as cholesterol, is unlikely to harm and may even enhance health. However, after cholesterol becomes oxidized by processing, it can become integrated into the endothelial lining of coronary blood vessels, cause free-radical damage to the vessel, and begin the formation of an atheromatous plague. This may, in turn, eventually impinge on the vessel lumen, cause clot formation, reduce blood flow to the heart muscle, and result in angina or even a life-threatening heart attack (see Figure 21-4).

The more toxic fat our bodies contain, the greater the chance for disease and the less chance to enjoy the health benefits derived from natural-form essential and nonessential lipids.

The dynamic and complex aspects of fatty acid chemistry help us to understand nutrition at a more meaningful level. Percent fat on a food label is essentially useless in determining the healthiness of a product. Instead, the following questions are more relevant to health:

1. Are the fats saturated or unsaturated? Saturated fats are deposited into adipose tissue more readily than unsaturated fats. Saturated fats are more stable than unsaturated fats when cooked.
2. If the fats are unsaturated, what is the ratio of omega -9s to -6s to -3s? Omega -3 fatty acids and omega -6 linoleic fatty acids are oxidized by the

body more readily than are omega -9 oleic fatty acids.[1] Higher omega -3:6 ratios are more natural and more healthy.

3. Have the fats been hydrogenated? If so, what are the levels of potentially toxic *trans-* isomers?

4. Are the lipids oxidized from exposure to air and light or complexed with other nutrients, such as protein, which occurs in high heat processing?

5. What is the length of the fatty acid chain? Long-chain triglycerides (more than 12 carbons long) are readily deposited in fat reserves, whereas medium-length chains (eight to 12 carbons long) are more readily utilized for body energy.[2]

6. Does the product contain the nutrients that were associated with the lipid in its natural context, such as antioxidants, vitamins, and minerals?

7. What is the stability when the fat is subjected to time, heat, light, and air?

8. How have the fats degraded in processing?

9. In a processed product, how have the lipids been stabilized? No antioxidants — worst; synthetic antioxidants — better but still bad; natural antioxidants — best.

Percent fat or number of calories doesn't answer questions of health

(For resources of natural antioxidants to use in cooking and products incorporating the above principles, see page 263, no. 4.)

---

1. Storlien, L.H. "Not all dietary fats may lead to obesity." The American Journal of Clinical Nutrition 51 (1990): 1114.

2. Senior, J.R. Introductory remarks by Chairman. In *Medium Chain Triglycerides*. Philadelphia: University of Pennsylvania Press, 1968.

Obesity has created an economic heyday. Consumers seeking quick and easy fixes and instead become easy prey for entrepreneurs.

Self-sufficiency is not profitable

A free-enterprise, market-driven, capitalistic society creates constant economic opportunity. Corporations, individual enterprises, and professionals self-servingly attempt to create a dependent mindset within the public. Our being convinced that we need professional services and products to properly survive and achieve the "good life" makes a good life for others. Self-sufficiency, individuality, and prevention do not create as much revenue opportunity, and thus are either ignored or not promoted by a society that measures its worth in terms of its gross national product.

Complex problems are believed solved with purchases

Various pharmacologic agents have been developed which attack obesity in parts of its cycle. They are all band-aids and, at best, can give only short-term results. They ignore the synorgonic nature of obesity and should not be relied upon as long-term solutions.

This is not to say that a short-term application of some of these agents in conjunction with efforts to achieve the Synorgon Diet may not be helpful in some instances. For those individuals who are at imminent risk from continued obesity, pharmacologic agents may provide an only recourse. But be fully aware that they all have potentially serious side effects and should be used only with extreme caution and as a last resort.

Examples of these pharmacological approaches include appetite suppressants such as amphetamines (Dexedrine, Obetrol, phentermine, Fastin, fenfluramine, Pondimin, and several others).

Treatments for obesity often exacerbate the cause of obesity – imbalance – by creating more imbalance

Another category of pharmacologic agents is the absorption inhibitors. These are designed to decrease the absorption of dietary carbohydrates and lipids. They include drugs such as Acarbose and AO-128, an alpha-glucosidase inhibitor; phaseolamin from kidney beans, which inhibits the action of pancreatic amylase on carbohydrate digestion; sucrose polyesters; and others.

Other examples include thermogenesis enhancers such as caffeine, nicotine, and ephedrine; digestive coaters; and non-absorbable food materials such as the new fat substitutes, synthetic sweeteners, and a host of other clever compounds.[1-4]

Most interventions treat imbalance — which obesity is — with more imbalance. Such methods attempt to force a complex biological system into compliance by myopically addressing single mechanisms. In the long term it can be predicted, and in the short term it has been found to be true, that such interventions bring far more potential for danger than good.

The logic of enzyme blockers, for example, would suggest that obesity occurs because

Surgical treatments address results, not causes

people digest carbohydrates. But carbohydrate digestion is essential for life. Stomach coaters would suggest that obesity results from absorbing food components. But the absortion of food components is necessary for life. The use of synthetic fat substitutes would argue that absorbtion of natural fats is unhealthy. But this is untrue since certain amounts and kinds of fats are esssential for survival. When these treatments are given, imbalance can indeed occur, such as when fat substitutes hold fat-soluble essential nutrients within the lumen of the digestion track, not permitting their absorption, and thus potentially resulting in fat-soluble vitamin deficiencies.

Surgical interventions represent even more egregious examples of the silver-bullet approach to complex problems of balance.

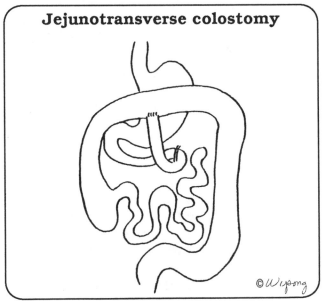

Jejunotransverse colostomy

©Wysong

Figure 22-1

Lipectomy is the surgical removal of fat stores, usually through suction. It may solve the result of obesity but it will not curtail the accumulation of fat. Jaws have been wired shut to prevent eating.[5] The stomach has been stapled (gastroplasty) to create a smaller lumen and more rapid fill.[6,7] The stomach may be wrapped with Teflon® so it cannot distend.[8] The stomach, jejunum and ileum can be surgically bypassed to prevent ab-

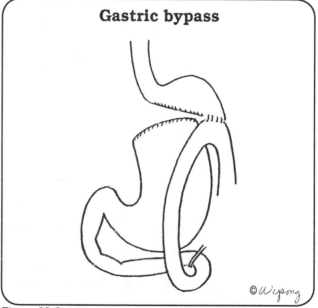

Gastric bypass

Figure 22-2

sorption of ingested foods.[9,10] Balloons have been inserted into the stomach to create an artifical sense of fullness.[11] And the vagus nerve has been severed to interfere with the neural control of eating and digestion.[12]

Although such procedures are recommended only when all else fails and an individual is over 100 percent overweight, they

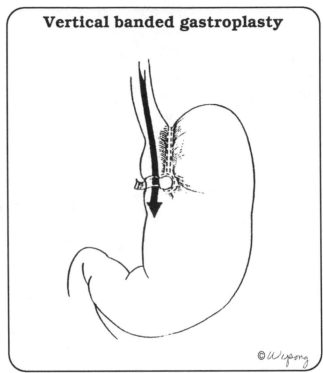

Vertical banded gastroplasty

©Wysong

Figure 22-3

are performed with increasing frequency early
in obesity.   Additionally, these procedures
have a high rate of complications. The mortality rate for jejunoileostomy, for example, is
5 percent. The morbidity (health complica-
tion) rate is appreciable in all these procedures, as is true of any surgical intervention
in the obese. The difficulty of having to work
through several inches of fat, the poor access
to surgical sites, the tendency for ligatures to
slip or tear tissue, the slippery instruments
and greasy gloves are well known by all
surgeons.   Then, even if surgical success
occurs, the patient may succumb to
atelectasis (collapse of the lung), pneumonia,

wound infection, dehiscence (breakdown of wound tissues), and thromboembolism (blood clots).

Many surgical obesity procedures are later reversed, more than doubling the rate of morbidity and mortality. Second surgeries may involve a nutritionally and emotionally compromised patient and increased surgical risk working with remodeled, scarred, inflamed, and perhaps infected tissue that is also less healthy and resilient.

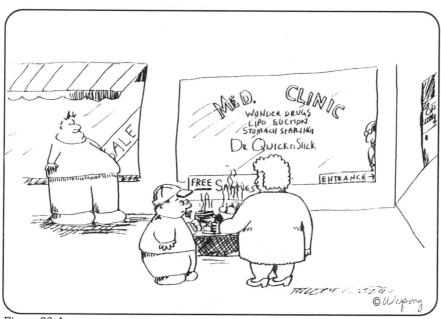

Figure 22-4

Dietary programs range all the way from total fasting to the use of prepared meal substitutes; from the consumption of single foods such as grapefruit or popcorn to various forms of calorie counting and balancing of protein, fats, and carbohydrates.

Fasting or starvation diets result in loss of muscle mass, decreased endurance, mood swings, sleep disturbances, cold intolerance, loss of energy, increased susceptibility to disease, and general degradation of the quality of life. Dangers from starvation diets also include ketosis, depressed thyroid and adrenal hormones, electrolyte imbalances, cardiac dysrhythmias, hyperuricemia, hyponatremia, hypokalemia, hypoglycemia, neutropenia, alopecia, and renal loss of phosphate and magnesium.[13] Prolonged weight loss decreases the levels of omega -3 fatty acids, the beneficial immune stimulating and health enhancing fatty acids discussed in Chapter 21.[14] Fasting can also lower the metabolic setpoint and increase the efficiency of food assimilation, storage, and use, so that when the diet is broken more weight is gained back than was there originally (as discussed in Chapter 17).[15]

Novelty diets, such as eating only grapefruit or bananas and skimmed milk, can often result, predictably, in a deficiency of certain nutrients, setting the stage for susceptibilty to disease.[16]

A preoccupation with excluding fat from the diet can also create imbalances. Very low calorie diets with less than one gram of fat can cause biliary stasis (bile stoppage) and resultant gallstones. Increasing fat to 10 grams, as would be at least a minimum found in the natural synorgonic diet, would avoid this problem.[17]

Perhaps the most popular current dietary regime is known as the protein sparing modified fast. These diets are characterized by high protein and low fat contents. They are designed to conserve lean muscle mass while forcing the burning of fat stores. When first introduced, they used a low-quality collagen protein source, and by 1977 more than 60 deaths had resulted. The newer diets have been redesigned and are of higher biological value. They are reported to be both safer and more effective.[18] Some such diets have also reportedly been effective for non-insulin-dependent diabetes mellitus.[19] But high-protein diets can result in kidney problems as well as decreased thyroid function.[20] Additionally, if fats are rapidly metabolized out of body stores, ketosis can result if there are not sufficient carbohydrates available to metabolize the acetyl CoA in the citric acid cycle. The brain will not function well on ketones, and large amounts of water are necessary to dispose of the ketoacids generated from the rapid metabolism of body fat stores.[21]

Protein sparing diets are usually in the form of commercial preparations which mix into meal-substitute drinks. A review of the ingredients in these formulations usually shows a dramatic departure from natural foods. A representative list of ingredients is presented in Figure 22-5. This composition more closely resembles something synthesized in a chemist's laboratory than that grown in a farmer's field. Such dietary products, even if they do create weight loss, should be held under high suspicion because they depart from natural synorgonic balances and may result in long-term consequences. It should also be said that follow-up studies of protein sparing and very-low-calorie diets do not show them to be effective in terms of long-term weight maintenance.

Typical Diet Drink Ingredient List

Sucrose	Sodium Chloride
Soy Protein Isolate	Ascorbic Acid
Calcium Caseinate	Ferrous Fumarate
Cellulose Gum	Niacinamide
Gum Arabic	Vitamin A Palmitate
Carboxymethylcellulose	Zinc Oxide
Pectin	Calcium Pantothenate
Guar Gum	Manganese Sulfate
Oat Bran	Thiamine Mononitrate
Corn Bran	Phytonadione
Maltodextrin	Cupric Oxide
Artificial Vanilla Flavor	Pyridoxine Hydrochloride
Fructose	Vitamin D_3
Aspartame	Riboflavin
FD & C Yellow No. 5	Folic Acid
FD & C Yellow No. 6	Vitamin B_{12}
Potassium Chloride	Chromium Chloride
Dibasic Calcium Phosphate	Biotin
Magnesium Oxide	Sodium Molybdate
Titanium Dioxide	Potassium Iodide
Vitamin E Acetate	

Figure 22-5

Predictably, radical diets, drugs, and surgery are not solutions. Sorry, but what has taken 200 years since the beginning of the industrial era to foul up, is not going to be fixed in a morning on the surgery table or in a month by simply taking a pill.

Quick-fix interventions miss the point and ignore the fundamental problem of synorgonic imbalance.

1. Vertes, Victor, M.D. "Obesity in America." Complementary Medicine 2 (Jan./Feb. 1987): 9.
2. Council on Scientific Affairs. "Treatment of Obesity in Adults." The Journal of The American Medical Association 260 (1988): 2547.
3. Pi-Sunyer, F. Xavier. "Obesity" in *Modern Nutrition In Health and Disease*. Philadelphia: Lea & Febiger, 1988, p. 807.
4. Ibid, 809.
5. Ibid, 812.
6. Vertes, Victor, M.D. "Obesity in America." Complementary Medicine 2 (Jan/Feb. 1987): 9.
6a. "Surgical Means of Weight Reduction." Complementary Medicine 2 (Jan./Feb. 1987): 26.
7. Pi-Sunyer, F. Xavier. "Obesity" in *Modern Nutrition in Health and Disease*. Philadelphia: Lea & Febiger, 1988, p. 812.
8. Ibid.
9. Ibid, 811.
10. Ibid, 812.
11. Moody, Frank G., M.D. "Surgical Management of Morbid Obesity." The New England Journal of Medicine 318 (1988): 387.
12. Pi-Sunyer, F. Xavier. "Obesity" in *Modern Nutrition in Health and Disease*. Philadelphia: Lea & Febiger, 1988, p. 812.
13. Newmark, S.R. et al. "Survey of very-low-calorie weight reduction diets: II. Total fasting, protein-sparing modified fasts, chemically defined diets." Archives Internal Medicine 143 (1983): 1423-1427.
14. Hudgins, Lisa Cooper and Hirsch, Jules. "Changes in abdominal and gluteal adipose-tissue fatty acid compositions in obese subjects after weight gain and weight loss." The American Journal of Clinical Nutrition 53 (1991): 1372.
15. Drenick, E.J. et al. "Weight reduction by fasting and semi-starvation in morbid obesity: Long-term follow-up" in *Obesity: Comparative Methods of Weight Control*. Westport, Conn.: Technomic Publishing Co., Inc., 1980, p. 25-34.
16. Council on Scientific Affairs. "Treatment of Obesity in Adults." The Journal of The American Medical Association 260 (1988): 2549.
17. Klawansky, Sidney, M.D. and Chalmers, Thomas C., M.D. "Fat Content of Very Low-Calorie Diets and Gallstone Formation." The Journal of the American Medical Association 268 (1992): 873.
18. Council on Scientific Affairs. "Treatment of Obesity in Adults." The Journal of The American Medical Association 260 (1988): 2548.

19. Usitupa, Matti I. J. et al. "Effects of a very-low-calorie diet on metabolic control and cardiovascular risk factors in the treatment of obese non-insulin-dependent diabetics." The American Journal of Clinical Nutrition 51 (1990): 768.

20. Turner, Lori Waite, M.D., R.D. "Very-low-calorie diets." Nutrition Clinics 4 (Jan./Feb. 1989): 3-5.

21. Ibid, 4.

Section II

What You Need
To Do

23 - GUIDELINES INTRODUCTION

We have extracted ourselves from our environmental synorgonic roots. Restoring health to our lives will mean reestablishing natural archetypal balances. Understanding our natural heritage, our genetic context, provides a broad rational principle for designing a healthful life. Read and reread Chapter 1 until this principle is firmly implanted in your mind and will.

The philosophic direction provided by looking to our genetic roots is the key to lifelong health success

But a beautiful principle is twice flawed: it is always imperfect, and its pure application is impossible to achieve. Similarly, divided highways and stop signals, in principle, should prevent auto accidents. But they don't. Similarly, the Synorgonic Diet provides a sound rationale and reliable road map, perhaps imperfect, perhaps not always easily followed, but nonetheless solid direction that can produce lasting results.

Our world's complexity and our feeble understandings of it do not make for easy black and white, right and wrong decisions. But getting ourselves pointed in the right direction is a good start. From there we will find ups and downs and many grey areas, but general progress can be achieved. An ideal life will not occur overnight and may not occur in a lifetime, given the pressures of modern society. However, steady, sure, significant enough progress can be made to improve weight and to reap the health and vitality benefits that can result.

*The
solution
to obesity
requires
funda-
mental
lifestyle
and
attitude
changes*

Achieving and maintaining normal weight is a challenge because the solution to obesity is involved, requiring lifestyle and attitude changes. Our human tendency is to simply leave things as they are. Inertia is a powerful force preventing improvement. Particularly is this so because change is often uncomfortable. And losing weight can be expected to be uncomfortable not only behaviorally, but physically — because our bodies have established their own physiological inertia. With this understood, efforts should not be abandoned at the first sign of discomfort or inconvenience. Expect some difficulty and welcome it; it is a sign that you are on your way.

The beauty of the synorgon philosophy is that it provides guidance for most areas of choice. It helps to refine and sharpen our own intuitive sense of the right and wrong of natural law, if you will, rather than imposing some new, strange, and awkward thought and action pattern upon us. Eating whole, fresh, raw foods just plain feels right to the mind, whereas eating a diet food made primarily from synthetic chemicals does not. Reflection causes us to say, "I knew that" about fundamental truths, but to be suspicious and feel uncomfortable about irrational belief systems. Therein lies the utility of synorgonic rationale. It is not a fad, it is a powerful rational friend you can have for life.

The guidelines in the following chapters are not all encompassing. They need not be. Armed with the synorgon philosophy, you will be able to derive some of your own ideas for action. Additionally, you will be able to intelligently sort through the constant barrage of diet gimmicks, products, and programs. Use this as a rule of thumb: Any program is doomed to failure if it simply promotes a product or a radical departure from a natural diet, rather than education and assistance in making fundamental changes that balance life's activities and restore synorgonic dietary patterns.[1]

Applying the understanding of the Synorgon Diet, you are on your way to being self-determining. But remember, food and lifestyle decisions are not always reducible to right or wrong, black or white, but rather to better or worse. Don't expect perfection, but always press toward the ideal.

---

1. Turner, Lori Waite, M.S., R.D. "Very-Low-Calorie Diets." Nutrition Clinics 4.1 (Jan./Feb. 1989): 11.

Although it is true that how we look outside is usually a reflection of our physiological appearance (health) within, this is seldom the reason weight loss is pursued. Instead, we become preoccupied with appearance for its sake alone. This can lead to impulsive, superficial, and poor choices. Obesity is a health problem. If you feel unattractive, understand that this is simply a by-product of health improperly cared for. Correct the health problem and physical attributes will improve. Magic-bullet weight reduction methods address only appearance, the facade, the window dressing of obesity, not its substance, its core problem...poor health.

Throw your scale and skin-fold calipers away. Forget about body fat; think about health. Learn about your body and its nutrition by reading, questioning, and listening. Seek ways to optimize health. Be determined to stay young, disease free. (Subscribe to the monthly *Wysong Review* newsletter empowering people in personal, social, and planetary health, listed on pages 258 and 263, no. 2.)

Review Chapter 6 on the health consequences of obesity. This list should be as sobering as the list of diseases caused by smoking. Though some people respond to fear, it is not always a prime mover. Take the positive approach and seek health, not absence of disease.

Make it a career. Health is life's truly great treasure. Lose it and you'll agree. Take charge. Get informed but never assume your limited knowledge totally defines the world. Stay humble, ever learning. Eating and living for best health can take care of weight automatically.

25 - CHANGE SHOULD BE GRADUAL

A long-term result is worth patience. Cycles of starvation – hoping for immediate results – and then over-rewarding or even just eating what you ate prior to the diet, ultimately result in net weight gain (see Chapter 17).

It took approximately 200 years to transform our world into its modern, synthetic, technological mode, which has put us out of sync with our natural environmental context. We were born into this new artificial world and so were our parents. Thus there is a strong personal pull, a familiarity, camaraderie and comfort, if you will, with this new synthetic world. It will thus require considerable reorientation, even though our genetics are tuned to a natural world quite unlike our present circumstances.

Obesity is a chronic condition. Chronic conditions result in sweeping physiological, biochemical, and anatomical compensations. The body, with time, tends to view these new compensations as normal, as a new set point, and thus any effort to change them is met with resistance and even discomfort. It is important to understand that a chronic condition, such as obesity, requires a chronic long-term effort to cure and restabilize the body to its normal healthy weight level.

Attempting a radical change often requires dramatic behavioral changes that the brain simply cannot sustain. The discomfort experienced from an effort to dramatically change weight can be likened to the agony of withdrawal from addicting drugs (see Chapter 11).

Also consider that not everyone will be able to lose weight at the same rate. It is also not important that everyone lose the same amount of weight. A person 60 years old who has osteoarthritis of the knees and hips as a result of the stress of carrying excess weight may greatly benefit from the loss of 25 to 30 pounds, even though that person may be 100 pounds overweight. Attempting to strip off more weight will meet with increasing metabolic resistance and may be so discouraging that effort may be stopped, and even the initial 25 to 30 pounds regained.

In contrast, a young woman in her early 20s would be well advised to continue with the diet until the entire 100 pounds is lost, because the effort to achieve this weight costs far less than the consequences that can result over a lifetime of obesity.

Keep in mind that the initial rapid weight loss that occurs when embarking on a low-calorie dietary program cannot be sustained. The initial weight lost is in part adipose tissue, but it also is glycogen and associated water (see Chapter 17). After the glycogen and water are lost, weight loss slows down remarkably. If a person does not understand this mechanism, he may easily become despondent and no longer continue his efforts (see Chapter 16).

Another physiological reason for slow weight loss is that, under certain conditions, fluid can be retained masking weight loss for up to 16 days even though fat is being lost through dieting. Additionally, individuals with undiagnosed or untreated thyroid disease and those on medications that lower energy expenditure may lose weight very slowly.[1]

On average, it is necessary to keep caloric intake to approximately 1,200 kilocalories per day. This will result in a loss of approximately two pounds of adipose tissue a week. A person will thus consume approximately 1,200 kilocalories per day less than the average 2,400 kilocalories energy expenditure.

As discussed throughout this book, the Synorgon Diet, however, does not rely upon the mathematics of calorie counting. The above simply is meant to describe what can and cannot be expected. These caloric targets can be achieved by modifying the diet to whole natural foods and adjusting lifestyle as described in the synorgon program.

The accompanying chart shows a desirable rate of weight loss (see Figure 25-1). An average loss falling between the two lines would mean approximately 80 pounds lost in a year. Notice the rapid weight loss in the beginning as a result of the depletion of glycogen and water.

Be sure not to be so aggressive with a dietary program that weight loss occurs greater than that described by the upper line. If this occurs, imbalance can result and dietary failure becomes more likely. Also consider that if this line is exceeded, lean body mass will be lost more rapidly. If this happens, metabolic rate will decrease, weight loss will become more difficult, and weight gain will be more efficient.

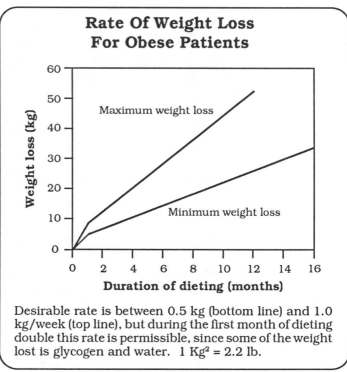

Rate Of Weight Loss For Obese Patients

Desirable rate is between 0.5 kg (bottom line) and 1.0 kg/week (top line), but during the first month of dieting double this rate is permissible, since some of the weight lost is glycogen and water. 1 Kg² = 2.2 lb.

Figure 25-1

1.   Newburgh, L.H. and Woodwell, Johnston M.   "Endogenous obesity - a misconception." Ann. Intern Med. 3 (1930): 815-825.

26 - GET SMART; USE FORESIGHT

As discussed in Chapter 19, a child — or an animal for that matter — simply reacts to moment-by-moment pleasure and pain stimuli. In the wild, such behavior, which relies primarily on instinct, is appropriate and can assure survival.

But human intelligence has added a new factor in the equation of survival. Our ability to dramatically disrupt our environment requires us to use the same intelligence which is capable of such manipulation to judge long-term consequences by the use of foresight. Similarly, we teach our children the long-range value of education, of not eating sweets constantly, of limiting television watching, of appropriate social behavior, and so forth. We instruct them because we can intelligently project consequences.

But look at the reasons we use to decide to diet. The primary concern for women is appearance, shortness of breath, and poor exercise tolerance. For younger women it is infertility and for older women it is pain in the back, hips, and knees. On the other hand, men seek health when they begin to experience angina from heart disease or they are refused life insurance at normal rates.[1] Notice that none of these reasons employs the use of foresight.

The use of intelligent foresight is required because reward and punishment are not going to be immediate. We must make adjustments even though we may never truly discern a direct cause and effect relationship.

For example, the fatty acid composition of the membranes that enclose all body cells can be adversely altered by a diet laden with oxidized fats and hydrogenated oils. Evidence abounds in the literature demonstrating that such changes in tissue will ultimately result directly or indirectly in disease. But it can take three to four years to change those fatty acids in membranes to natural fatty acids that have not been adversely altered from food processing. Obviously, it is not going to be possible to immediately feel the results of, for example, deleting all hydrogenated oils from your diet.

Thus the changes that need to take place for healthy weight maintenance require intelligent foresight. This is not to suggest that it is easy, but anyone can do it. The problem is complex, similar to that of mastering a foreign language. It is difficult, it requires time, but anyone can do it if he/she is diligent enough.

Remember, our minds got us into our present predicament. We must use our minds, our unique ability to project consequences, to get us out.

---

1.   Garrow, J.S. "Treatment of obesity." The Lancet 340 (1992): 409.

27 - BALANCE SYMPATHETIC AND PARASYMPATHETIC ACTIVITIES

Seek pleasurable activities that are not associated with eating (see Chapter 11). Such activities stimulate the creative and active sympathetic senses. Exercise, sports, nature-related activities, satisfying social relationships, finding new, challenging and productive forms of work, or making sure that in your present vocation you give 100 percent — these all qualify.

Become socially or environmentally active. Find a good cause, such as protecting a wildlife habitat, or preventing pollution, or local philanthropic or social programs. Get excited and throw yourself into it. The pleasure from such activities will help replace some of the excess pleasure that was received from parasympathetic eating and leisure...and calories will be burned in the process.

---

28 - SEEK HEALTHY COMPANIONS

Remember how we wanted to be just like the prettiest or the most athletic boy or girl in school? Use envy and peer pressure to your advantage. Seek friends and groups who challenge you by their healthy lifestyle and appearance. When we choose friends who have the same problems as ourselves, we risk excusing our own inadequacies and seeing abnormal as "normal."

In athletics, if you only compete against those who are equal or inferior to you, you will not improve. Not only will you not improve, but your skills will actually decline. On the other hand, playing against superior athletes will cause you to rise to the occasion and improve. Use this principle to win the weight game.

Good associates are those who understand natural nutrition, self-care, and environmentalism, and are intellectually alert and socially responsible. Join organizations with synorgonic kinds of agendas and befriend those you wish to emulate.

------

29 - MAKE EXERCISE A PART OF EVERYDAY LIFE

Activity can make a difference just as it did for our "wild" ancestors who were never obese. A typist simply switching from a manual to an electric typewriter can add two pounds of fat per year by the energy saved. Increasing opportunity for ease in daily life must be offset by committed efforts to be more active.

Walk or bicycle to work, or other locations normally driven to. Begin a garden in the yard. Plant trees in vacant areas. Repair and upgrade the home yourself, rather than hiring it done.

Engage in an exercise program that will result in continuing challenges. Perform a wide range of exercises incorporating aerobics and resistance training, and keep a log on how much time is spent on each exercise, how much weight is used in each set, how much time between sets, and how many repetitions are performed. This permits focusing on goals and attempting to achieve continuing progress.

Endless variations of exercises are possible. The best are those that encompass the entire body engaging multiple joints. Functional exercises, those that mimic real life body movements, such as stair climbing, squats, deadlifts and bench presses, are more effective than isolated exercises such as "Thigh Master" exercises or seated leg extensions.

Regardless of the exercise, it must continually challenge you. Increasing repititions, increasing weight, increasing exercise sets (repititions of certain exercise) and decreasing rest between exercises are the ingredients for dramatic body and health improvements. Don't overdo it, however. Thirty minutes two to four times weekly with one or two days rest in between will do wonders and decrease the chances of injury, exhaustion or boredom. On days off, stretch, walk and keep low-intensity active.

Join a health club, subscribe to fitness magazines, find a workout partner who helps push you. Befriend someone you would like to look like. Study that person's routine, emulate it and determine to equal or surpass him or her.

Use models to achieve the body you desire. A soft, fat, saggy body is that of someone who sits, lies, and occasionally walks. The body actually starts to look like an overstuffed chair. If that's the body you want, then that's what you do. On the other hand, a very lean, more cardiovascularly fit body is that of the distance runner. If you distance run, that's what you could look like. A more muscular, lean body is that of the sprinter. Increased muscle tone results from weight lifting with moderate weights and higher repetitions. More massive muscular size results from lifting higher weights with low repetitions and lots of rest in between. Pick the body you want by picking the exercise.

Without exercise, weight lost is two thirds fat and one third lean tissue (primarily muscle). The more lean tissue lost, the lower the resting metabolic rate and the harder further weight loss becomes. Exercise, particularly weight bearing, can help prevent the loss of this calorie-burning lean muscle.

Incidentally, it is a misconception that male weight lifters will become muscle bound or that female weight lifters will look like the heavily muscled, narrow-hipped, small-breasted body builders in magazines. Such bodies result from practically obsessive full-

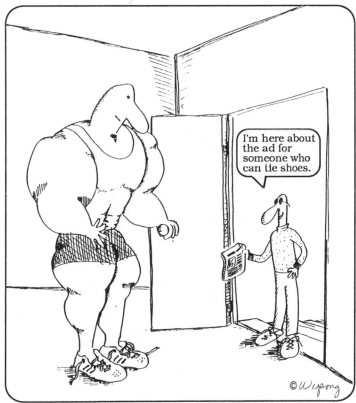

Figure 29-1

time dedication to lifting and usually (but seldom admitted) the use of anabolic steroid drugs.

Robust exercise will create body shaping both inside and out. How you look outside is a reflection of how you look inside. The lifestyle that creates a soft flabby weak outside makes a soft flabby easily-diseased inside. A lean muscular, strong athletic outside reflects a strong resistant inside as well.

Don't set limits on your capabilities, but strive to be the very best it is possible for you to be. Don't set a time limit on it, either. Determine to be an octogenarian or even nonogenarian athlete.

A challenging progressive exercise program puts more focus on who you are physically. A renewed spirit and a commitment to progress escalate as progress is made. In addition to this, of course, exercise burns calories, increases lean tissue mass and raises metabolic rate, helping to dissipate fat stores as well as efficiently metabolizing fats. Stationary bikes and treadmills will not, however, negate the unhealthful effects of poor dietary patterns.

Regardless of the exercise program you choose, work into it gradually and don't expect results overnight. Make a lifetime commitment to fitness activity. Gradually increase the challenges, try new variations and work out with friends to prevent boredom. With time, patience, and perseverance, you will begin to look like the goals you have set. The physical and mental reward of having a fit body will more than pay for the effort. An excellent program for fitness is to alternate weight lifting with aerobic exercise — walking, biking, running, swimming, and such sports as basketball, volleyball, soccer, etc. (or try the undiscovered fun and fitness challenge of competitive badminton! - see Chapter 14).

Regardless of the activity, you must use the principle of progression and overload to bring your body to a new fitness height. Your metabolism — your structure — will change only if you send the message to it through physical challenge that it must improve. This requires effort, sweat, and even perhaps a little discomfort. If you do only what is easy, that means your present body is adequate and will thus not change.

Don't believe those who tell you to take it easy and not exert yourself. Nothing in life, other than disease and death, is easy.

30 - TAKE TIME TO EAT

Eat in a relaxed atmosphere and don't bolt down food boluses with drinks. Anxiety and stress do not encourage proper digestion or the proper functioning of satiety mechanisms. Digestion begins in the mouth with chewing and salivary enzymes and should be given the opportunity to do so. A good rule of thumb is chew your drinks and drink your food. Don't rinse food with beverages but let sufficient chewing create the liquid that is swallowed. Food should be chewed until there is nothing more to chew.

Train yourself to eat slowly and thoroughly. Try to eat alone. No television, no radio, no reading, no gabbing. Just you and

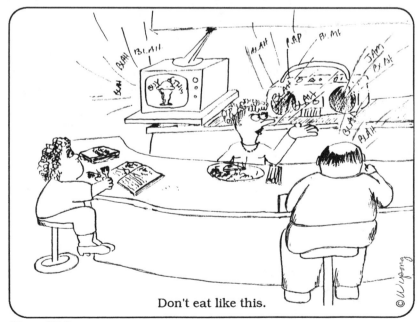

Don't eat like this.

Figure 30-1

your food. Concentrate on each mouthful. Make it your objective to thoroughly dissolve both solids and liquids in saliva before swallowing. When eating under other circumstances, your "alone training" can be recalled as a reminder to slow down and eat thoroughly.

Taking undistracted time to eat will increase the nutritional value of what is eaten and create earlier satisfaction, thus decreasing the amount consumed.

———————————

31 - CHANGE THE NUMBER OR SIZE OF MEALS

Work toward reducing meals to twice daily with no snacks other than fresh fruit. There is decreased utilization of food and increased calorie expenditure if infrequent meals are eaten. Our bodies are not designed to consume food almost continually during waking hours, as is now possible. In the wild, the norm was more infrequent meals with little opportunity for snacking. Digestive organs need rest, as do other organs. The constant barrage of food, much of which is demanding to digest, is likely the cause of the universal pancreatic hypertrophy common in animals and humans on overdoses of processed, enzyme-devoid foods. Pancreatic exhaustion, cancer, diabetes, and obesity may be the eventual result.

Pancreatic Size

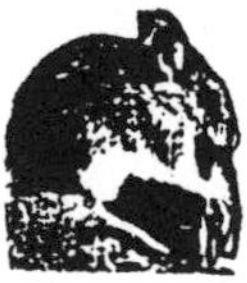

Pancreas % of
Body Weight

Wild Mice 0.32%
Laboratory Mice
  on Processed Foods 0.84%

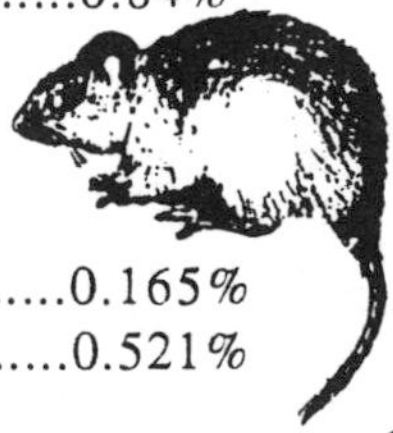

Rats on a Raw Diet 0.165%
Rats on a Processed Diet......................0.521%

Figure 31-1

The thermogenic (calorie burning) effect of meals is greatest in the morning and least (causing weight gain) in the evening.[1] The following is one example of a schedule which uses this principle.

Early morning
1. Fresh fruit, or
2. Fresh squeezed fruit juice, or
3. Fresh squeezed juice with mixed-in barley or wheat grass powder, spirulina, or blue-green algae alternated on different mornings. (For sources, see page 263, no. 3.)
4. Combined with the following supplements:
   • Probiotic powder
   • Food derived antioxidants A, C, E (For sources, see page 263, no. 3.)

Mid to late morning
(when hungry — largest meal of the day)
1. Bowl of alternated whole-grain properly cooked cereals with rice or soy milk or dairy with yogurt. (For proper cooking technique and sources for organic grains and milk, see the May 1992 *Wysong Review*, page 7.) Combine with:
2. Dried or fresh fruit as sweetener (For sources, see page 263, no. 3.)
3. Soaked chopped raw nuts (For proper technique and source, see page 263, no. 3.)
4. Fresh flax seed oil (For source, see page 263, no. 3.)
5. Enzyme, vitamin and mineral supplements (For sources, see page 263, no. 3.)

Afternoon
> Fresh fruit and vegetables only

Late afternoon
> Supper, using synorgonic principle (see next section on food combining)

Late evening
(if hungry — but try to avoid since food eaten in the evening is most likely to be deposited as fat)
> Fresh fruit, oil-free, air-popped popcorn or baked oil-free snacks (For sources, see page 263, no. 3.)

---

1.   Romon, Monique, et al. "Circadian variation of diet-induced thermogenesis." The American Journal of Clinical Nutrition 57 (1993): 476.

Food variety is important...but not necessarily at the same meal. For example, the body's need for balanced amino acids can be met by eating different amino acids at different meals. Also, consider the demands on the digestive organs of a meal containing wine, pop, salad oil, ice water, lettuce, carrots, lobster tail, potatoes, melon, onion soup, white rolls, pecan pie, and ice cream. (When could this ever occur in the wild?) Try mixing these all together in a bowl. To sort and separate all these complex foods into retrievable nutrients is an incredible task we are asking of our body, considering each food has its own digestive demands. Little wonder our organ systems become prematurely exhausted and we become diseased and aged prematurely. Indigestion often results, foods are wasted by simply passing through to be then fermented into gas in the bowel, and cravings rather than satiety result. Simpler meals (varied from meal to meal) with fewer foods, well chewed, will increase food efficiency and satisfaction.

Some general rules of thumb:
1. Eat fruits alone. Most can be combined but melons are best eaten alone, or at least first.
2. Meats should be eaten first. (Remember to try for more and more meatless meals.)
3. Fresh or steamed vegetables can be eaten with any meal except fruit.

4. Eat any high-fat food last.
5. Make meals a simple combination of one class of foods requiring cooking, with steamed or fresh salad. For example:
   - grains plus veggies only
   - meats plus veggies only
   - potatoes or other tubers plus veggies only
   - legumes plus veggies only
6. Eat out less. If eating out, eat salads first before ordering anything else. This will quell your enthusiasm for a four-course meal and may be satisfying by itself. Otherwise order ala carte using rules 1-5 above. Don't be afraid to ask restaurants to cater to your needs. If they won't, eat elsewhere.

———————————

33 - EAT PORTIONS AND LEAVE SOME

Fill a plate and don't get seconds – except for raw vegetables, if desired. We often take the Mount Everest approach to eating: Why did we eat it? Because it was there.

Leave some on your plate when finished. Food left is cheaper and healthier than food deposited as fat.

Don't sit at the table when done, looking at filled serving bowls. Get away from the table, brush your teeth (we hesitate to redirty a clean mouth), and engage in some activity. Light exercise such as walking, house or shop work or stretching is a good idea and seems to assist digestion and refocus our attention away from the kitchen.

Make it a personal goal and challenge to not eat unless hungry, and stop when you're enjoying it the most.

Remember the powerful force of our eating "on" switch, and vow to control it (see Chapter 13).

------

34 - EMPHASIZE COMPLEX CARBOHYDRATES

Whole vegetables, fruits and grains well chewed can create much satisfaction, in contrast to rich, refined, sugary, and fatty foods which promote continual cravings. Natural-form carbohydrates moderate blood sugar levels and provide a clean, efficient fuel for mental and physical tasks (see Chapter 12). In contrast to fats and proteins, complex carbohydrates burn cleanly to water and carbon dioxide, and there are no known dangers to their consumption.

Consume fiber-rich foods. Whole, natural foods contain appropriate levels of both soluble and insoluble fiber. If fiber-depleted foods are used, then fiber supplementation, in moderation, should be incorporated with such meals. But if fiber supplements are taken, drink six-eight glasses of water a day (see Chapter 15).

Use grains in variety. Try cereals or side dishes made from quinoa, buckwheat groats, basmati rice, amaranth, spelt, millet and others. (For techniques and sources, see page 263, no. 3.) Learn how to sprout seeds for salads, cereals and sandwiches. (See page 263, no. 1.)

Ideal synorgonic sources of fiber would be those foods that can be eaten raw. Fruits, vegetables, and sprouts would therefore be most nutritional. Grains, legumes (beans, soy, peanuts, etc.) tubers (potatoes) and other vegetables requiring cooking to be digestible would be second choices since many nutrients are destroyed by heat.

No, you will not be protein-starved. Does a horse, cow, hippo, or elephant look protein starved? All vegetation has protein and, when eaten in variety, it can provide the essential nutrients.

---

35 - REDUCE FLAVORS

Our taste buds, not our health, are the target of a gigantic processed food industry. In a recent issue of Food Technology, the monthly journal of the Institute of Food Technologists, approximately 500 advertisements appeared in 350 pages. Of the hundreds of ads for ingredients and processing technology, not one addressed primarily nutrition and health. Instead, they focused on taste.

With such extraordinary technology and skill manipulating our palate, we don't have a prayer. A recent issue of the British Medical Journal, the Lancet, drew the conclusion that obesity in large part is due to the high palatability of our recreational foods.[1]

Modern foods are designed to practically compel us to crave them and to eat them...lots of them.

Natural whole real foods are by contrast somewhat subtle in flavor, even bland, permitting our gustatory senses to select foods based on the nutritional needs our inner voice calls for. Once these foods are fractionated into pieces and parts and then dyed, perfumed and embalmed, our inner senses become dulled and confused. Wholesome natural foods, the foods we need for health, become boring. Similarly, a child taken to a carnival every day will soon become bored with his wooden rocking horse at home.

Some condiments stimulate appetite and cause overconsumption. Some will create cravings long after the stomach is stuffed. Foods too hot or too cold may also create cravings.

Salt intake should be moderate. High insulin levels found in obesity tend to conserve sodium.[2] Additionally, refined commercial salt is of questionable safety and also creates cravings and excess consumption. Use a truly natural, unprocessed, trace-mineral-rich salt. (For sources, see page 263, no. 3.)

Use whole, fresh, natural foods at moderate temperatures as much as possible. With time, the subtle flavors of nature will be fully statisfying.

Read books and subscribe to magazines which emphasize natural cookery. The delightful variety of healthy eating awaiting you will change your senses, sharpen the discernment of your nutritional palate and will soon make your former flavor-supercharged foods objectionable. (For sources, see page 263, no. 1.)

---

1. Bradley, P.J. "Pathophysiology of obesity." The Lancet 340 (1992): 848.
2. DeFronzo, R.A. et al. J. Clin. Invest. 58 (1976): 83-89.

36 - CONVERT TO WHOLE, FRESH, RAW FOODS

If this simple obvious thing were done it is unlikely that anyone would be able to accumulate or sustain excess body weight. The ideal goal is to move the diet ever more toward whole, fresh, raw, natural foods. It is, in fact, all you have to do with your diet to achieve healthy weight. Even high-fat raw foods, such as avocados and nuts, will not cause obesity.

Processed refined foods, such as sugars, syrup, oils, fried foods, etc., create cravings that are difficult to control. The assumption that natural foods are unflavorful and boring is incorrect. The palate will readjust and delight in the new kaleidoscope of subtle varieties of flavors in natural foods and will no longer require tastebuds to be flooded with sugars, white paste, grease, and spices.

Incidentally, if pregnant, don't even think about feeding your baby the champion of all junk foods, formula. The weight gained in pregnancy is specifically to support nursing. If you don't nurse, you keep the weight, and the baby gets experimented on.

The additional benefits of nursing include resistance to breast cancer and, a child with a higher IQ and better health including decreased risk of obesity.[1]

Feeding infant formula under the illusion that it is "100% complete and balanced" is like feeding pets "100% complete and balanced" packaged foods. For a glimpse of this disaster (thousands of pets have died), and as a warning against buying into the mythology that nutritionists know 100% about nutrition, see Appendix IV.

---

1. Wysong, R.L. *Wysong Review*. Wysong Institute: Midland, MI, 1993, Vol. 4, Tape #6, Vol. 6, No. 9, and Vol. 6, No. 11.

37 - SEEK FOODS RICH IN NATURAL MICRONUTRIENTS

If the brain is not supplied the raw material to synthesize neurotransmitters (see Chapter 12), the mental chemistry necessary to support your new diet and lifestyle will not be possible. In their whole state, fruits, vegetables, nuts, and whole grains are excellent micronutrient sources, and should be incorporated as much as possible into the diet.

More exotic, but extremely rich nutrient sources include flower and bee pollen, kelp and other seaweeds, spirulina and blue-green algae, barley and wheat grass juice or powder, and a host of herbs. (For sources, see page 263, no. 3.)

A wide range of helpful publications can help design meals based on natural nutrient dense foods. (For sources see page 263, no. 1.) You will find that it is a misconception that the only satisfying and tasteful foods are those that are deep fried, processed, meat based, or from a fast-food outlet.

Fat natural raw products are important nutritionally, but are exceedingly dangerous once a food has been processed and packaged. As discussed in Chapter 21, light, heat, and various minerals and chemicals within foods once ground and mixed together can cause the degradation of food lipids. The more nutritionally valuable the lipid is, such as essential fatty acids, the more vulnerable it is to degradation from processing.

Lipids within processed foods, once degraded and then consumed, can displace nutritional fatty acids within the body's structure and metabolism. Over time, this can result in serious disease consequences.

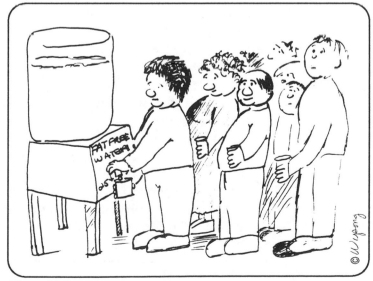

Figure 38-1

Additionally, once lipids are degraded, they can in effect become toxins such as the oxidized forms of fatty acids and cholesterol, resulting in a wide range of diseases including atherosclerosis and heart disease.

If oils are on the ingredient label of a packaged product, be sure that they are not hydrogenated or partially hydrogenated oils. Oils that are more stable to processing include various saturated fats such as butter, palm and coconut oil. Other stable oils include the high oleic sunflower oils, olive oil and canola oil. But again, it is best to try to find packaged foods to which no oil has been added. (For resources, see page 263, no. 3.) Avoid deep fried foods. If they are consumed, be sure to remove all of the fatty breadings and crusty coatings before consuming whatever is left inside. It's interesting to see the heap of greasy coating piled on your plate in contrast to the amount of real food you dug out of the middle. When you look at this pile, ask yourself whether it is best left there on the plate or should be in your stomach — an easy question, you'll see.

Fats can virtually drench processed foods. Manufacturers know that fats and oils increase mouth feel and palatability and thus do what they can to assure your repeated purchases. Try to increasingly avoid all processed foods and home prepare your own meals and lunches. This will put you in more control of your own health and weight destiny.

———————

39 - CONSUME OPTIMAL TRACE MINERALS AND VITAMINS

Any fresh natural food is a bountiful source of micronutrients. Mill, freeze, retort, dry, extrude, flake, and puff — and "poof" these micronutrients are gone. Every processed meal that is eaten must draw on body reserves for the micronutrients necessary to process and utilize the food. Since obesity results in large part from the consumption of processed foods, the obese are far in debt and micronutrient starved.

Sea vegetation, such as kelp, dulce, spirulina and blue-green algae are rich sources of such trace minerals. The iodine contained in these sources may also help stimulate thyroid activity, which is often depressed in the obese.[1]

Multiple vitamin and mineral supplements may ensure against deficiencies that could lead to cravings. Seek sources made from real foods. (For resources, see page 263, nos. 3 and 4.) Additionally, pollen, barley, wheat grass, yeast, figs, other fresh and dried fruits, and nuts are excellent whole food sources of vitamins and minerals. (For resources, see page 263, no. 3.)

In addition to converting the diet to more and more fresh whole foods, try to incorporate some of the more exotic nutrient-dense foods mentioned on page 204.

---

1. Benum, Sara. "Feast or Famine, An Examination of Weight Management Issues." *Complementary Medicine* 2.3 (Jan./Feb. 1987): 10.

40 - RICH, NATURAL SOURCES OF OMEGA -3 FATTY ACIDS SHOULD BE INCREASED

Omega -3 fatty acids are found in many foods, particularly in flaxseeds, soybean, and rape (canola) seeds, as well as in many species of fish and animals. It is interesting, as well as being a verification of the wisdom of the Synorgonic Diet, that wild meat, dairy and eggs contain much higher levels of the health-enhancing omega -3 fatty acids than their factory-farmed counterparts.

Omega -3s can help curtail the autoimmune activity possibly present in obesity, and counteract the imbalance of omega -6 fatty acids commonly found in today's diet (see Chapters 8 and 21). Additionally, omega –3s are known to decrease insulin resistance.[1] Even though they are a lipid, omega -3s are considered anti-obesity nutrients (see Chapter 21).[2]

If fresh, whole vegetables and fruits are emphasized in the diet, the dietary fat profile will be ideal to increase fat calorie oxidation, supply essential fatty acids, and decrease fat deposition. Some fats are more slowly used for energy, and therefore are more likely to lead to fat storage. These include: long-chain saturated fats, common in animal products; and linoleic acid, which predominates in corn and other common grain sources. On the other hand, omega -3 fatty acids and short- and medium-chain fatty acids are oxidized readily, augment the immune system, and are least likely to be deposited in fat reserves (see Chapter 21).[3]

---

1. Storlien, L.H. et al. "The type of dietary fat has a profound influence on development of insulin resistance in rats." Diabetes Res. Clin. Pract. 5 (suppl. 1): S267 (abst.).
2. Cunnane, S.C., et al. "Essential fatty acids decrease weight gain in genetically obese mice." Br. J. Nutr. 56 (1986): 87-95.
3. Leyton, J. et al. "Differential oxidation of saturated and unsaturated fatty acids in vivo in the rat." Br. J. Nutr. 57 (1987): 383-393.

41 - RESTORE THE ENVIRONMENT

We are not isolated and insulated from the rest of the world. We are an inextricable part of synorgon. If synorgon is disrupted, how can we expect to survive? We therefore must change our myopic focus from self to synorgon.

Try to reestablish a natural nontoxic environment in the home, workplace, and world. Set the heat down. This alone can cause you to increase calorie burning. Think purity in terms of water, air, food, and land, and become active in its restoration and preservation.

Focusing on what we can do to clean and restore our natural synorgonic context will automatically lead to better personal life choices. (For resources on what you can do for the environment, see page 263, no. 1.)

Use the synorgon philosophy in all life choices and not only your health, but the Earth's will be improved. Walk or bike to work, don't drive. Use the stairs, not the elevator. Grow your own organic garden. Make your yard organic. Plant trees. Make a wildlife habitat. Help clean a river; stop industrial pollution. Doing all these things is the Synorgon Diet in action.

I know this can all seem far afield from your weight loss problem, but it is not at all. It in fact adresses the core obesity cause: our removal from synorgonic content.

---

42 - LOSE WITHOUT DIETING

Using the more accurate (see Chapter 9) net caloric figures for fat (nine calories per gram) and protein and carbohydrate (three calories per gram), it becomes apparent how weight reduction can occur without dieting.

The normal 2,500-calorie food intake for adults consists of about 40 percent fat calories and weighs about one and a third pound (611 grams).

If you consume the same amount of food (611 grams) but reduce its fat content from 111 grams (40 percent of calories) to 34 grams (15 percent of calories) by increasing calories from carbohydrate and protein, the total calories for the day would decrease from 2,500 to 2,038. But the food intake would be the same. The difference, 462 calories per day, represents an incredible difference in fat that would have been put on the body or fat that could be lost...about 40 pounds in a year. And, again, it was done without dieting, and by eating just as much food and getting just as full.

If whole, natural, vegetable-based foods are primary in the diet, you will automatically achieve 15 percent or less of calories as fat, because it is rare that natural foods contain more than this. When you purchase packaged foods, a simple calculation can be made to be sure the product qualifies for 15 percent or less. Multiply the grams of fat on the label

How To Lose Without Dieting

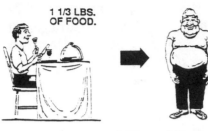

40 pounds of fat
in a year.

A Normal Day's Food

111 gms. fat...1000 calories (40%)
500 gms. protein / carbohydrate.......................................1500 calories(60%)
Total = 611 gms. (1 1/3 pounds)...2500 calories

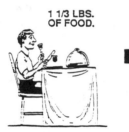

Healthy
weight maintenance.

Eating the same amount of food but reducing fat.

34 gms. fat..307 calories (15%)
577 gms. protein / carbohydrate..1731 calories (85%)
Total = 611 gms. (1 1/3 pounds)...2038 calories

Net daily fat avoided: 462 (2500 - 2038) calories / day

- 3% thermic loss =

448 net calories per day ✕ 365 days =

163,520 calories per year ÷ 9 calories / gm (fat value) =

18,169 gms. ÷ 454 gms. (pound conversion) =

40 lbs. of fat avoided per year

Figure 42-1

by nine and divide the result by the total calories listed on the label. For example, if the label reads three grams of fat and 100 calories, 3 grams x 9 = 27 calories ÷ 100 calories = .27 (27 percent) of calories are fat (see Figure 42-2).

A Bad Buy

NUTRITIONAL INFORMATION
SERVING SIZE .... 1/2 cup, 4 oz.
SERVINGS PER CONTAINER....... 3-3/4
CALORIES.................................... 100
PROTEIN...................................... 4.25 g
CARBOHYDRATE.......................... 13.75 g
FAT.. 3 g
CALORIES FROM FAT................. 27
SODIUM....................................... 320 mg
POTASSIUM................................. 480 mg

Figure 42-2

Appetite and digestion altering drugs should be avoided if at all possible (see Chapter 22). Such drugs avoid causes, delay needed fundamental changes, and always pose risks.

Some medications, however, may be necessary until appropriate modifications in diet and lifestyle can be made. For example, diabetes should be controlled since it is a strong appetite stimulant and is almost always associated with obesity. Don't blindly stop any and all medications and simply begin drinking carrot juice and munching on nuts. Be patient. Consult with qualified professionals (nutritionally-oriented holistic practioners preferably) as necessary (see Resource 263, page 1).

Get ever more informed and move slowly and surely in the right direction. With time, hopefully all medications can be avoided and you will be in synorgonic balance on your way to a life of health and healthy weight.

There are some more natural aids without the more serious side effects of pharmaceuticals which some have found helpful on the road back to healthy weight. I call these crutches since they are not the solution but are simply an assist to help you get back on the road.

• Ginger – Ginger is an herb which has been widely used for motion sickness, colds, flu, digestive problems, and irregular menstruation. A recent study showed that its warming effects increased thermogenesis (the burning of calories while at rest) and may assist in dieting.

The best ginger is fresh. Obtain recipe books to learn how you can incorporate ginger into your meals.[1] (For Resource, see page 263, no. 1.)

• Tryptophan – Tryptophan is an amino acid which was recently used quite widely for sleep disturbances and for its calming effects. A byproduct of its use was that it helped decrease fat tissue.

Unfortunately, this amino acid has been removed from the market because a bioengineered form had caused serious side effects in some users.

Tryptophan is, however, quite abundant in pumpkin seeds. By consuming up to six or seven ounces of pumpkin seeds, some have reported that appetite was significantly curtailed for several days.[2]

• Arginine and carnitine – These amino acids may assist in weight reduction by, in the first case, increasing levels of growth hormones and, in the second case, by transporting fat across mitochondrial membranes for oxidation. These amino acids are available in local pharmacies or health food stores. Follow the dosage recommendation of the manufacturer.

• Chromium – Chromium is a trace mineral that assists in the metabolism of sugars. It forms part of a biochemical complex called "glucose tolerance faster," and it enhances the effects of insulin. Taken daily at 200-400 micrograms, chromium has been found to increase fat loss and preserve muscle. This increases metabolic rate and thus speeds calorie burning. Other beneficial effects include lowering elevated blood sugar and decreasing appetite, especially for sweets.

Chromium is deficient in the diet of most people.[3] It is a part of many broad spectrum vitamin and mineral products.[4] For resources see page 263, no. 3.

• Ephedrine/caffeine combinations –Danish researchers have found that by combining 20 milligrams of ephedrine with 200 milligrams of caffeine three times a day, that significant weight loss can occur while lean muscle mass is preserved.

One physician recommends taking Sudafed, a form of ephedrine, in 30 milligram tablets, combined with 200 milligram tablets of No-Doze, a caffeine source. This approximates the 20-200 milligram combination used by the Danish researchers. This combination can be taken once or twice daily after breakfast and lunch.

Some people will experience some tremors or nervousness, but these initial side effects will decrease over time.[5]

Again, a reminder. These are temporary crutches. Use them only if you reach a sticking point and use them only intermittently. The main emphasis of your efforts should be achieving Synorgon Diet and lifestyle balances.

---

1. Wysong, R.L. *Wysong Review*. Wysong Institute: Midland, MI, 1993, Vol. 7, No. 1.
2. Wysong, R.L. *Wysong Review*. Wysong Institute: Midland, MI, 1993, Vol. 7, No. 2.
3. Anderson, Richard A. et al. "Breast milk chromium and its association with chromium intake, chromium excretion, and serum chromium." The American Journal of Clinical Nutrition 57 (1993): 519.
4. Chromium manufacturers: Nutrition 21, 1010 Turquoise Street, Suite 335, San Diego, CA 92109 (619) 488-1021; and Inter Health, 1365 N. Broadway, Suite 100, Walnut Creek, CA 94596 (415) 930-6300.
5. Astrup, Arne. "Pharmacology of thermogenic drugs." The American Journal of Clinical Nutrition 55S (1992): 246.

44 - DIET FOR ONE DAY

The reason most diet programs fail is not only because they do not address fundamental synorgonic problems, but because people simply tire of counting calories or being regimented to costly meal replacements day in and day out.

But anyone should be able to muster up the willpower to diet for one day.

The program is as follows: You can eat anything you want one day but you must diet the next day. This cycle simply continues until you can properly adjust your eating patterns to the Synorgonic Diet. It has the psychological advantage of giving you an objective you can achieve — dieting for only one day.

During the diet day you are free to eat all the fresh fruit you desire. You can also eat micronutrient-dense foods such as spirulina, barley and wheat grass juice powders, blue-green algae, and whole food antioxidant and micronutrient supplements. (For Resources, see page 263, no. 3.) Fresh-squeezed fruit and vegetable juices diluted with purified water can also be consumed and used to mix with the above powders.

The day you are not on the diet you are free to eat anything you want, if that is what you need for proper motivation. If possible, however, on the non-diet day, try to convert the diet more and more to healthy foods and synorgonic balance. Also try to drink one to two glasses of water one half hour before each meal.

By dieting just one day, the metabolic rate does not drop as it does in very-low-calorie starvation-type diets, and thus fat continues to burn. Eating fruits, micronutrient-dense foods, and a specially-designed nutriet supplement that helps curb cravings on the diet day helps you maintain blood sugar levels, build nutritional strength, and detoxify. (For Resource, see page 263, no. 3.)

The net weekly calorie (especially fat calories) intake will decrease because you simply will not be able to make up for the deficit of the diet day in the next day. (Granted you actually could, but you would need to eat the equivalent of two days' food in one day...a real pig-out orgy.)

45 - CONCLUSION

Most weight management programs provide a variety of specific recipes. This one hasn't. If I give you a recipe and you don't like it or you get bored with daily menus I describe and therefore don't lose weight, you might thumb your nose at the whole book.

Hopefully the bigger recipe, the recipe for living, the philosophy described here will be palatable — it can be — but it is up to you to work out the particulars that will work best for you. The basic guide that the diet — and daily living for that matter — should be restored to its natural balances is an easy concept. It can serve as a filter for decision making and puts you in the driver's seat. Lifestyle and menus can be devised which work for you, are flexible, and can thus be tailor made to be a part of the rest of your life.

Most recipe books have merit and can be adapted to fit synorgonic archetypal patterns. Whole grains can replace white flours, whole fruits can replace juices or sweetners, most fats and oils as isolated ingredients can be eliminated, and fresh salads can replace vegetables from a can. The principle is easy. The more your food looks like what could be picked in a garden, the better it is for you. Being perfect in this regard is not the point. Forward progression in the right direction is.

Similarly, lifestyle patterns can be made more archetypal. Getting daily fresh air and

sun, exercise, play, walking, and running;
becoming challenged by work; being determined to succeed; and contributing to making this a better world are goals within reach
of all of us. The principle is easy. The more
your life reflects the various physical and
mental challenges which would be present if
you were to fend for yourself in the woods,
the better that life is for you.

Thinness is not an appropriate goal in
and of itself. Gaining it through starvation or
a pill at the expense of good health is a poor
exchange. What is the difference between
these follies and cutting forests, strip mining, oozing effluent, or belching exhaust to
simply increase profit, luxury and ease?
Physical and economic narcissism must give
way to an Earth and health ethic. Indeed,
seeing ourselves as an integral part of something bigger changes our focus to the
whole...that is the essence of the synorgon
philosophy and the Synorgon Diet. If we care
for the world around us, benefits return to us
in terms of lasting health and even appropriate weight.

Armed with the knowledge that each of
us is an inextricable part of a larger whole, a
new awareness and sensitivity emerges. We
no longer see ourselves as simply consumers, opportunists, capitalists, or hedonists.
We become touched by a universal ethic of
synorgonic fiduciary responsibility, foresight,
caring, nurturing, and protecting. The Earth
becomes an extension of our bodies and our
bodies an extension of the Earth.

Our increasing care for the world we will leave to our children is not unlike the care we must extend to our own bodies. Polluting the body is like polluting the Earth. Squandering Earth resources is like squandering the vitality of our own lives. An Earth rightly cared for has the potential for boundless and paradisaic gifts. A body rightly cared for provides the potential for a long, healthy, vital, and productive life enjoyed more fully with a fit and trim body. The exciting and boundless benefits possible by achieving these synorgonic goals must be a preeminent focus for us all.

Please feel free to write to me in care of the publisher with questions or with your experiences in applying the Synorgon Diet.

Good health to you.

Appendixes

APPENDIX I - LIPID BIOCHEMISTRY

From *Lipid Nutrition: Understanding fats and oils in health and disease* by Dr. Randy L. Wysong, Inquiry Press, 1990.

FATTY ACIDS

Fatty acids, the basic building blocks of fat, are long-chain carboxylic acids, that is, hydrocarbon (alkyl) chains containing a terminal carboxyl (-COOH) chemical group.

Fatty Acid Structure

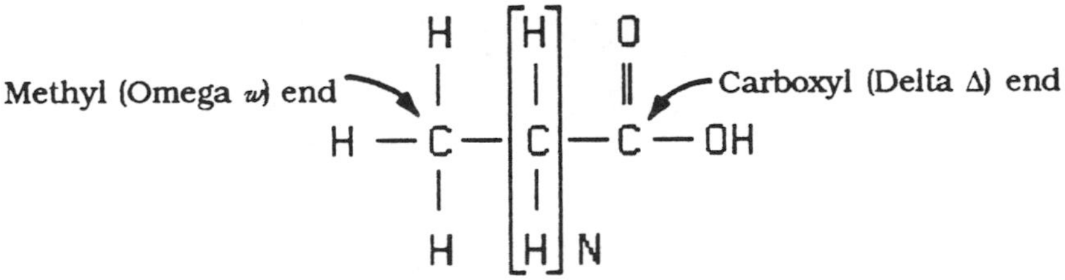

Methyl (Omega ω) end

Carboxyl (Delta Δ) end

N represents the number of repeating CH_2 units that vary with each fatty acid. For example in stearic acid (18:0), N = 16.

From *Lipid Nutrition: Understanding fats and oils in health and disease* by Dr. Randy L. Wysong, Inquiry Press, 1990.

Figure I-1

Fatty acids contain from 4 to 22 carbon atoms. They can be saturated (having no double bonds in the carbon chain), monounsaturated (with one double bond in the chain), or polyunsaturated (with several double bonds in the fatty acid).

In nature, fatty acids occur linked, or esterified, to glycerol and hence are called glycerides. If in solid form, they are called fats; if in liquid form, they are called oils. One

223

fatty acid esterified with glycerol is a monoglyceride, two combined is a diglyceride, and three (the most common) attached to the glycerol backbone is a triglyceride.

There are three locations on the glycerol molecule on which fatty acids can esterify. Saturated fats (such as palmitic and stearic acids) exclusively fit in the 1 and 3 positions whereas unsaturated fatty acids can distribute randomly among the three positions on the glycerol backbone. A common configuration is thus a saturated fatty acid in positions 1 and 3 and an unsaturated fatty acid in position 2. (Figure I-2; note that each point of the schematic drawing of the fatty acids represents a carbon atom.)

Structure Of A Triglyceride

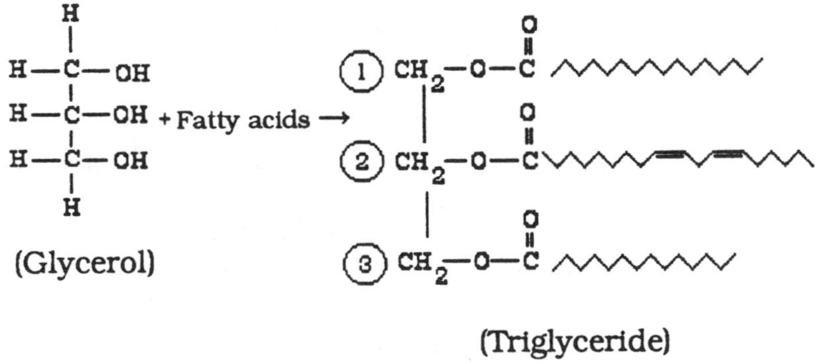

(Glycerol)

(Triglyceride)

Free fatty acids link (esterify) to glycerol to form triglyceride. The number one and three positions are usually occupied by saturated fats, whereas the number two position often holds an unsaturated fatty acid — such as linoleic acid ($18:2w6$) as seen here.

From *Lipid Nutrition: Understanding fats and oils in health and disease* by Dr. Randy L. Wysong, Inquiry Press, 1990.

Figure I-2

Both saturated fatty acids and fatty acids containing fewer than 16 carbon atoms are largely oxidized to provide energy. Fatty acids containing 16 to 22 carbon atoms can be oxidized for energy as well, but they can also be incorporated into cell membranes, regulate metabolism after conversion to eicosanoids (prostaglandins, thromboxanes, leukotrienes, lipoxins, and various other hydroxy analogs), changed to other fatty acids, or stored in fat (adipose) tissues.

Linoleic And Linolenic Acid Structure And Nomenclature

Linoleic acid (LA, 18:2w6)

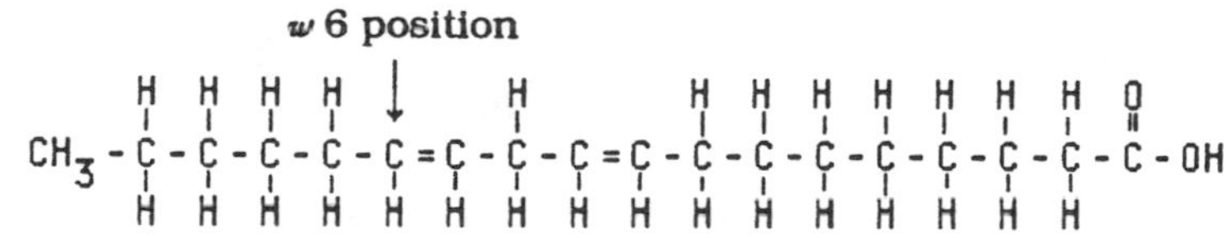

w 6 position

Linolenic acid (LNA, 18:3w3)

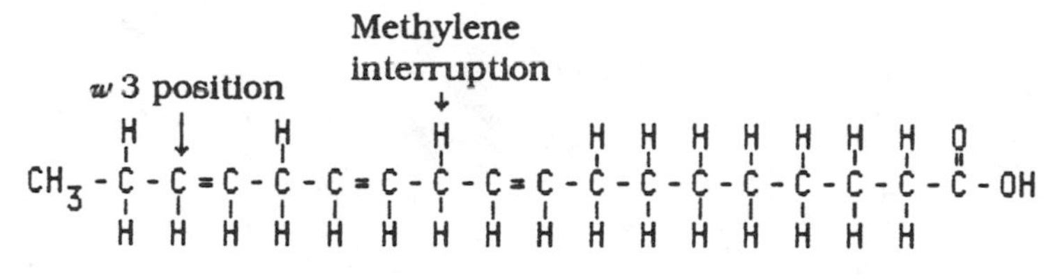

Methylene interruption

w 3 position

From *Lipid Nutrition: Understanding fats and oils in health and disease* by Dr. Randy L. Wysong, Inquiry Press, 1990.

Figure I-3

NOMENCLATURE

Abbreviated notations simplify fatty acid nomenclature. In the case of the notation for linoleic acid, abbreviated LA, 18:2w6, the 18

Nomenclature And Structure

NAME	ABBREVIATION	CODE
Butyric	BA	4:0
Caproic		6:0
Caprylic Acid		8:0
Capric Acid		10:0
Lauric Acid		12:0
Mysteric Acid		14:0
Palmitic Acid	PA	16:0
Palmitoleic Acid	POA	16:1 $w7$ cis
Stearic Acid	SA	18:0
Oleic Acid	OA	18:1, $w9$ cis
Elaidic Acid	EA	18:1, $w9$ trans
Linoleic Acid	LA	18:2, $w6,9$ all cis
Linolenic Acid	LNA	18:3, $w3,6,9$ all cis
Gamma Linolenic Acid	GLA	18:3, $w6,9,12$ all cis
Columbinic Acid		18:3, $w6$ cis,9 cis,13 trans
Stearidonic Acid	SDA	18:4, $w3$
Arachidic acid		20:0
Eicosaenoic Acid		20:1, $w9$ cis
Dihomo - ∂ linolenic Acid		20:3, $w6$, 9,12 all cis
Dihomocolumbinic Acid		20:3, $w6$ cis, 9 cis,13 trans
Eicosatrienoic Acid		20:3, $w9$, 12,15 all cis
Arachidonic Acid	AA	20:4, $w6,9,12,15$ all cis
Eicosapentaenoic	EPA	20:5, $w3$, 6, 9,12,15 all cis
Benhenic Acid		22:0
Erucic Acid		22:1, w 9 cis
Brassidic Acid		22:1, $w9$ trans
Docosahexaenoic Acid	DHA	22:6, $w3,6,9,12,15,18$ all cis

From *Lipid Nutrition: Understanding fats and oils in health and disease* by Dr. Randy L. Wysong, Inquiry Press, 1990.

Figure I-4

Of Common Fatty Acids
FORMULA

(BA) $CH_3 (CH_2)_2 COOH$

```
     H H H   O
      |  |  |   ⫽
H-C-C-C-C
      |  |  |   ⟍
     H H H   OH
```

$CH_3 (CH_2)_4 COOH$
$CH_3 (CH_2)_6 COOH$
$CH_3 (CH_2)_8 COOH$
$CH_3 (CH_2)_{10} COOH$
$CH_3 (CH_2)_{12} COOH$
(PA) $CH_3 (CH_2)_{14} COOH$
(POA) $CH_3 (CH_2)_5 CH=CH (CH_2)_7 COOH$
(SA) $CH_3 (CH_2)_{16} COOH$
(OA) $CH_3 (CH_2)_7 CH=CH (CH_2)_7 COOH$

```
     H H H H H H H H     H H H H H H H   O
      |  |  |  |  |  |  |  |      |  |  |  |  |  |  |    ⫽
H-C-C-C-C-C-C-C-C=C-C-C-C-C-C-C-C
      |  |  |  |  |  |  |        |  |  |  |  |  |  |    ⟍
     H H H H H H H     H H H H H H H   OH
```

(EA) $CH_3 (CH_2)_7 CH=CH (CH_2)_7 COOH$

```
     H H H H H H H H     H H H H H H H   O
      |  |  |  |  |  |  |  |      |  |  |  |  |  |  |    ⫽
H-C-C-C-C-C-C-C-C=C-C-C-C-C-C-C-C
      |  |  |  |  |  |  |        |  |  |  |  |  |  |    ⟍
     H H H H H H H     H H H H H H H   OH
```

(LA) $CH_3 (CH_2)_4 CH=CH CH_2 CH=CH (CH_2)_7 COOH$

```
     H H H H H H H H H H H H H H H H   O
      |  |  |  |  |  |   |  |  |   |  |  |  |  |  |  |    ⫽
H-C-C-C-C-C=C-C-C=C-C-C-C-C-C-C-C
      |  |  |  |      |          |  |  |  |  |  |  |    ⟍
     H H H H     H     H H H H H H H   OH
```

(LNA) $CH_3 CH_2 CH=CH CH_2 CH=CH CH_2 CH=CH (CH_2)_7 COOH$

```
     H H H H H H H H H H H H H H H H   O
      |  |  |  |  |  |   |  |   |  |  |  |  |  |  |  |    ⫽
H-C-C-C-C-C=C-C-C=C-C-C=C-C-C-C-C
      |  |  |  |      |          |          |  |  |  |  |    ⟍
     H H H H     H     H     H H H H   OH
```

(GLA) $CH_3 (CH_2)_4 CH=CH CH_2 CH=CH CH_2 CH=CH (CH_2)_4 COOH$
       $CH_3 (CH_2)_4 CH=CH CH_2 CH=CH (CH_2)_2 CH=CH (CH_2)_3 COOH$
(SDA) $CH_3 CH_2 CH=CH CH_2 CH=CH CH_2 CH=CH CH_2 CH=CH (CH_2)_4 COOH$
       $CH_3 (CH_2)_{18} COOH$
       $CH_3 (CH_2)_7 CH=CH (CH_2)_9 COOH$
       $CH_3 (CH_2)_4 CH=CH CH_2 CH=CH CH_2 CH=CH (CH_2)_6 COOH$
       $CH_3 (CH_2)_4 CH=CH CH_2 CH=CH (CH_2)_2 CH=CH (CH_2)_5 COOH$
       $CH_3 (CH_2)_7 CH=CH CH_2 CH=CH CH_2 CH=CH (CH_2)_3 COOH$
(AA) $CH_3 (CH_2)_4 CH=CH CH_2 CH=CH CH_2 CH=CH CH_2 CH=CH (CH_2)_3 COOH$
(EPA) $CH_3 CH_2 CH=CH CH_2 CH=CH CH_2 CH=CH CH_2 CH=CH CH_2 CH=CH (CH_2)_3 COOH$
       $CH_3 (CH_2)_{20} COOH$
       $CH_3 (CH_2)_7 CH=CH (CH_2)_{11} COOH$
       $CH_3 (CH_2)_7 CH=CH (CH_2)_{11} COOH$
(DHA) $CH_3 CH_2 CH=CH CH_2 CH=CH CH_2 CH=CH CH_2 CH=CH CH_2 CH=CH CH_2 CH=CH (CH_2)_2 COOH$

means the molecule has 18 carbon atoms, the 2 means that there are two double bonds in the molecule and the $w6$ means the first double bond begins with the sixth carbon atom counting from the methyl (CH_3), or omega (w), end of the carbon chain. The other end of the chain, the carboxylic acid (COOH) end, is termed the delta (D) end (see Figure I-3). Fatty acids are often represented schematically by a jagged line, where each peak and each trough represent a carbon atom in the fatty acid chain, as in Figure I-2.

PHOSPHOLIPIDS

Fatty acids with 16- and 18-carbon chains can participate in the manufacture of phospholipids which are the main structural components of cell membranes. Phospholipids are similar to triglycerides in that fatty acid molecules are attached to a glycerol molecule, a three-carbon alcohol or, less commonly, to sphingosine, a more complex amino alcohol. In triglycerides, all three esterifiable positions on a glycerol molecule are occupied by fatty acids. In contrast with phospholipids, the third position of the glycerol is esterified to phosphoric acid, which may in turn have other compounds attached to it, such as choline, serine, glycerol, inositol or ethanolamine (see Figure I-5). Lecithin, the best known phospholipid, has choline attached to the phosphate and is thus termed phosphatidylcholine. If phosphoric acid alone is attached, the compound is called a phosphotidate. Many molecular variations are also possible by mixing various fatty acids on the glycerol backbone.

Structure Of Phospholipids

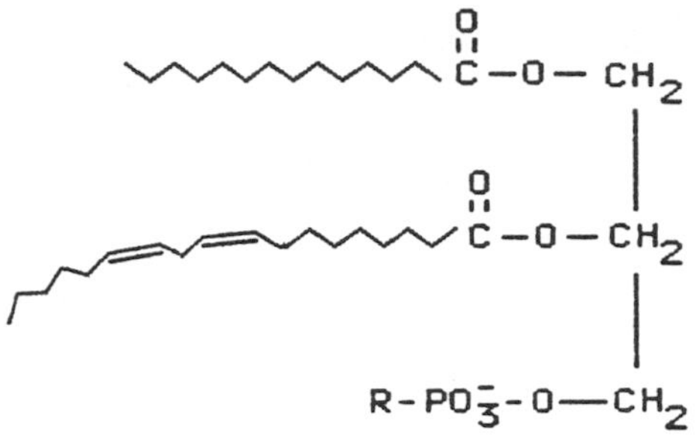

(R = Choline, serine, glycerol, inositol or ethanolamine)

A phospholipid in membranes usually has the phosphate attached to one of several different molecules (R). If R is choline, the molecule becomes lecithin (phosphatidylcholine).

From *Lipid Nutrition: Understanding fats and oils in health and disease* by Dr. Randy L. Wysong, Inquiry Press, 1990.

Figure I-5

ISOMERS

Fatty acid isomers have identical molecular formulas (the same numbers of each atom), but different chemical and physical properties. The two forms of fatty acid isomers are referred to as the cis- and the trans- forms, and can be distinguished from one another by the position of the hydrogen atoms on the carbons adjacent to the double bond.

Figure I-6 demonstrates these biochemically important forms of fatty acids. Notice that in the cis- form, the hydrogen atoms on the carbons next to the double bond are on the same side of the molecule.

The repulsive forces between these cis- "crowded" hydrogen atoms cause unsatur-

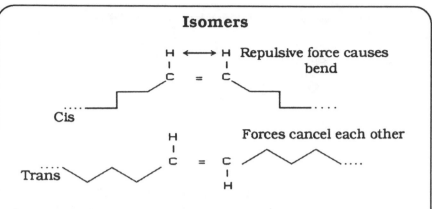

Isomers

Cis — Repulsive force causes bend

Trans — Forces cancel each other

The position of the hydrogen atoms adjacent to the double bonds creates different configurations of the fatty acid chain.

From *Lipid Nutrition: Understanding fats and oils in health and disease* by Dr. Randy L. Wysong, Inquiry Press, 1990.

Figure I-6

ated fatty acids to assume nonlinear (bent) shapes, which play an important role in lipid membrane configuration, fluidity, and biochemical reactions involving enzymes (see Figure I-7).

In the trans- form of fatty acids, the hydrogen atoms are on opposite sides of the molecule. Their repulsive forces cancel each other, leaving the molecule unbent. Although the trans- form is more stable, its chemical properties and biological functions are altered (see Figures I-6 and I-7).

BIOLOGICAL MEMBRANES

A biological (plasma) membrane only two molecules thick surrounds all cells as well as the organelles lying within the cell cytoplasm.

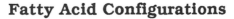

Fatty Acid Configurations

$\begin{matrix} O \\ \parallel \\ C \end{matrix}$ — OH   Stearic Acid
Saturated 18:0

$\begin{matrix} O \\ \parallel \\ C \end{matrix}$ —OH   Linoleic Acid
Trans-Unsaturated
18:2*ω*6

$\begin{matrix} O \\ \parallel \\ C \end{matrix}$ —OH   Linoleic Acid
Cis-Unsaturated
18:2*ω*6

Neck

Tail

Fatty acids can exist in rigid, straight configurations as in saturated and trans- forms, or in bent, more dynamic cis- forms.

From *Lipid Nutrition: Understanding fats and oils in health and disease* by Dr. Randy L. Wysong, Inquiry Press, 1990.

Figure I-7

Approximately one billion cells occupy the space of one cubic inch. To help visualize size: If we were the size of bacteria, a cell would be the size of a large auditorium housed by a skin two millimeters thick. The various drawings of biochemicals depicted in these pages would therefore be as they would appear from our size as bacteria — actually how we would see them through a giant magnifying glass.

The membrane is not a static sac, but rather a complex of chemicals with gates and pumps to control chemical and ionic balances, receptors for stimuli, and signal generators. This membrane is made up primarily of phospholipids, protein, and glycolipids. It is synthesized in situ (in the body) by components of food after they have been broken down by digestion.

Membrane lipids are amphipathic in that they contain both a hydrophilic, or "water loving," polar end and a hydrophobic, or "water hating," non-polar end. Phospholipids orient themselves into a bilayer sheet in membranes with hydrophilic ends pointed to the outside and the hydrophobic hydrocarbon tails pointing to the inside. (It is because of these properties that salts derived from fatty acids are important functional components of soaps, because their fat-soluble hydrophobic ends attract "fatty dirt" while their water-soluble hydrophilic ends can attract "watery dirt.")

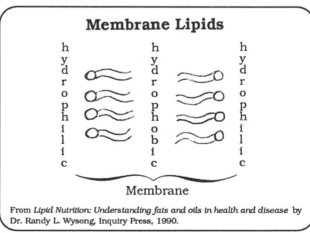

From *Lipid Nutrition: Understanding fats and oils in health and disease* by Dr. Randy L. Wysong, Inquiry Press, 1990.

Figure I-8

The neck of a fatty acid is located next to the delta (carboxyl) end and is stiff. The tail portion next to the omega (methyl) end, if containing cis- double bonds, is highly active, oscillating at a million vibrations per second (see Figures I-7 and I-9).

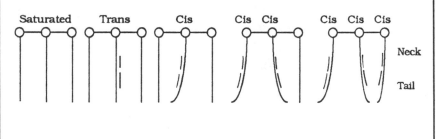

Triglycerides increase dynamic, metabolic and fluid properties as unsaturation increases and isomeric cis- form predominates.

From *Lipid Nutrition: Understanding fats and oils in health and disease* by Dr. Randy L. Wysong, Inquiry Press, 1990.

Figure I-9

Lipids, and some proteins within membranes, are also in constant lateral motion. In a bacterium, a single phospholipid will travel from one end to the other in one second. Thus, membranes are in effect two-dimensional dynamic solutions of an array of oriented molecules. Do you begin to see how complex and important dietary fats are? It gets even more remarkable.

Although membranes are considered lipid bilayers, there are other important components of the membrane. For example, almost 50 percent of the membrane is composed of protein, which serves many functional roles. In addition, the sugar residues of glycolipids (sphingosine + fatty acid + sugar: sphingomyelin for example) and glycoproteins (sugars attached to membrane proteins) protrude on the outer surface of membranes. Membrane fluidity is affected by cholesterol, and the length of fatty acid tails and their degree of saturation. Cholesterol sandwiched between membrane fatty acids prevents their crystallization (solidification) (see Figure I-10).

The specific spatial configuration (bent or straight) and electronegative discontinuity (charged on the data end, neutral on the other) of essential fatty acids permit linkage with sulfhydryl protein groups in membranes to form pi electron quantum mechanical membrane potentials that affect the transport of oxygen into tissues. Also, it is by means of the lipid membranes of mitochondria that cellular respiration occurs and energy is packaged for use throughout the body. Thus, dietary fatty acids, which ultimately build all membranes, indirectly affect the burning of nutrient fuels — the most fundamental of life's energetic properties.

Classic artists' renderings of biological membranes are overly simplistic and create an impression of static barriers. The real biological membrane is dynamic, containing millions of fatty acid tails vibrating at millions of times per second, with deletions, substitutions, and migrations in constant progress and biochemical doors opening and closing to permit the selective passage of food and waste. Biological membranes are more an action than a structure. Their complexity is literally beyond comprehension. It can be described with words, but not rationally fully grasped. Such is synorgonic reality.

Bilipid Cell Membrane

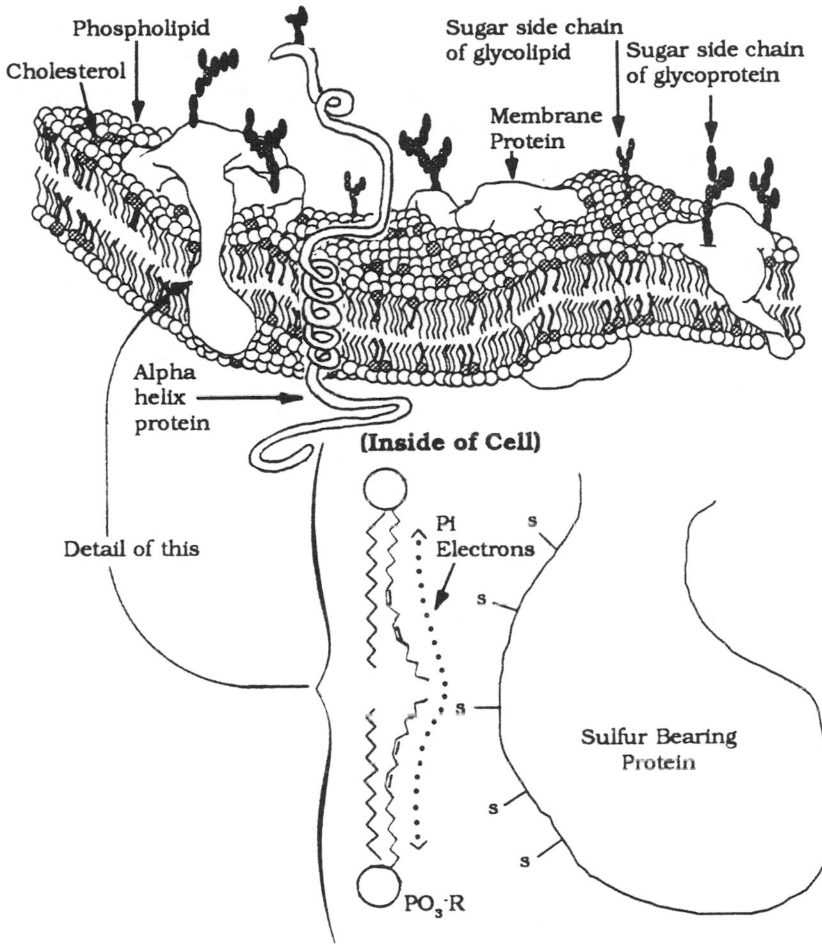

Phospholipids containing cis- essential fatty acids share pi-electrons with proteins to effect energy transfer through biological membranes.

From *Lipid Nutrition: Understanding fats and oils in health and disease* by Dr. Randy L. Wysong, Inquiry Press, 1990.

Figure I-10

When one considers that fatty acids comprise the membrane structure of all cells and their enclosed organelles, the breadth of the importance of dietary lipids begins to emerge. Membrane fatty acids are indeed the gatekeepers of life. (For further information on lipids in health and disease, obtain the book Lipid Nutrition, see page 262, no. ED050.)

APPENDIX II - LIPID DIGESTION

From *Lipid Nutrition, Understanding fats and oils in health and disease* by Dr. Randy L. Wysong, Inquiry Press, 1990.

To be deposited on the body, lipids must first be assimilated from the food. As the following brief outline shows, this process is very complex and again speaks to our theme of synorgonic interrelationships.

When a food is eaten, mastication helps separate the fats from the other components of the food. This permits digestion by digestive enzyme systems, which allow less than five percent of fats to pass undigested. In some species, including humans, digestion begins with the secretion by the serous glands on the back of the tongue, continues in the stomach with the action of gastric lipase, and is completed by pancreatic lipase excreted into the small intestine. As lipids enter the duodenum (the first part of the small intestine), hormones such as secretin and cholecystokinin are stimulated. These hormones influence lipid digestion by affecting the pH of the intestinal contents, the release of pancreatic lipase, and the secretion of bile.

More than 95 percent of fats eaten are absorbed

The increase in pH that occurs as the food mass, or bolus, moves from the acidic stomach into the duodenum is necessary to begin the fat-splitting activity of pancreatic lipase. Bile salts secreted from the liver emulsify the products of lipolysis (lipid breakdown), incorporating them into micelles, which are package complexes of bile salts, phospholipid molecules, and cholesterol (see Figure II-1).

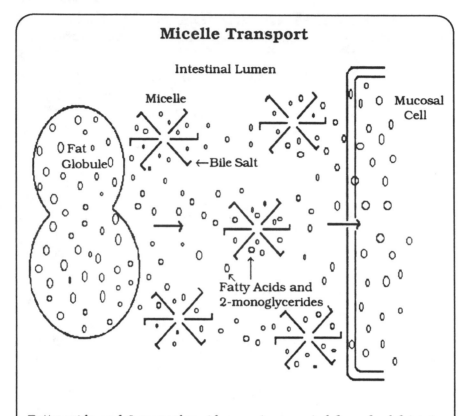

Micelle Transport

Intestinal Lumen

Micelle

Fat Globule

←Bile Salt

Fatty Acids and 2-monoglycerides

Mucosal Cell

Fatty acids and 2-monoglycerides are transported from food fat into intestinal cells by micelles which contain emulsifying bile salts.

Figure II-1

Fatty acid chain length determines the mode of digestion

Shorter-chain fatty acids complexed with the protein albumin can be absorbed both in the stomach and in the small intestine. Longer-chain triglycerides are disassembled in the small intestine by lipase, solubilized in micelles, and transported into mucosal cells (enterocytes) of the intestinal lining as free fatty acids, monoglycerides, and small amounts of glycerol, diglycerides, cholesterol, and phospholipids (see Figure II-2). After these components are in the mucosal

Lipid Absorption

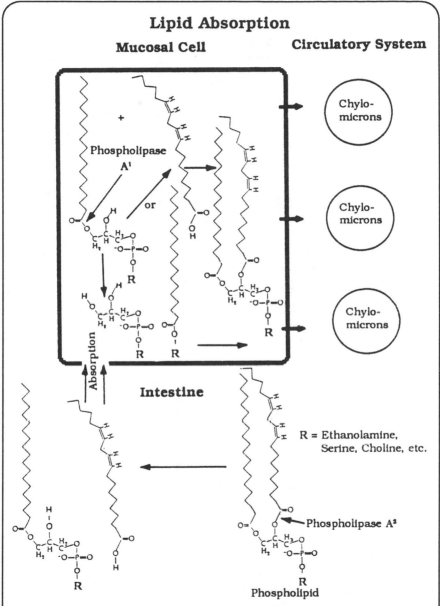

Lipids such as phospholipids are disassembled, absorbed into the intestinal mucosal cell, then reassembled and incorporated into chylomicrons to be transported within the body.

Figure II-2

cell, they are reassembled into triglycerides then corporated into chylomicrons, which are a type of lipoprotein that permits transport of lipids within the watery medium of the blood. The inner core of the chylomicron is composed of nonpolar ("water-hating") triglycerides and cholesterol esters, whereas the membrane is polar ("water-loving") and made up of phospholipids, cholesterol, and proteins, permitting solubility in blood.

Preparing lipids to survive in a watery body is exceptionally complex

Many intricasies of lipid digestion have been worked out in detail by researchers.[1-6] It is interesting to note that, in this process, the synorgonic principle of nothing working in isolation holds particularly true. The coordination of a variety of factors within both the food itself and the organism makes possible the delivery of lipids to organisms for energy, myriad metabolic processes, and the simple deposit of latent calories.

Fats are not simply consumed and then passively absorbed through the wall of the intestine. Rather, they are prepared by intricate emulsification systems, broken down in specific patterns by enzymes, absorbed by complex mechanisms, reassembled, and prepared for delivery to the body through complexing with a variety of other nutrients. These processes make it possible for non-water-soluble lipid components to be delivered efficiently throughout organisms that are comprised primarily of water; an incredible feat.

From this it can be seen that healthy function, which includes normal weight maintenance, requires the interplay of myriad factors and cannot be adequately addressed with simplistic, narrow-focused approaches. (For further information on lipids in health and disease, obtain the book *Lipid Nutrition, Undertanding fats and oils in health and disease*, see page 262, no. ED050.)

---

1. Barrowman, J.A. and Damton, S.J. Gastroenterology 59 (1970): 13-21.
2. Brockerhoff, H., et al. *Lipolytic Enzymes*. New York: Academic Press, 1974.
3. Moore, et al. Acta. Hepatogastroenterol 25 (1970): 30-36.
4. Hofmann, A.F. and Mekhigian, H.S. "Bile acids and the intestinal absorption of fat and electrolytes in health and disease." in *The Bile Acids*, Vol. 2, New York: Plenum Press, 1973.
5. Borgstrom B.Y. J. Lipid Res. 16 (1975): 411-417.
6. Dietschy, J.M., et al. Gastroenterology 61 (1971): 932-934.

APPENDIX III - ADIPOSE TISSUE

From *Lipid Nutrition, Understanding fats and oils in health and disease* by Dr. Randy L. Wysong, Inquiry Press, 1990.

Both the size and number of adipose cells can increase throughout life

The number of adipose (fat) cells in a human body can range from 2×10^{10} (20,000,000,000) to as high as 16×10^{10}.[1] That's a difference of 140 billion fat cells. There are thus tremendous potential fat reserves built into the body.

The size of an individual adipose cell can increase from 0.3 to 10 micrograms.[2] After cells are filled to maximum, they then increase in number. It is now believed that such increases in size and number can occur throughout life.[3]

Fat cells are formed from precursor cells called preadipocytes. After they are formed they do not dedifferentiate (change back) to their non-fat storing adipose cell precursors. Thus, after significant fat has been accumulated and adipose cell numbers increase, they remain eager to be filled as a fat memory bank, even if weight is later lost and adipose cells shrivel. Their presence increases the ease with which fat stores can be filled and weight can be regained. (The danger of gain and loss cycles is related to these cellular changes and is discussed in Chapter 17.)

Energy for biological functions in mammals can be derived from proteins, carbohydrates, or lipids. Other than in the liver, which readily converts amino acids to energy, amino acids derived from proteins are

242

conserved as much as possible to maintain muscle mass and the composition of a wide range of physiological biochemicals, such as enzymes. Normally, only during periods of starvation will the body begin to break down proteins to supply energy. On the other hand, sugars — either resulting directly from digestion or from the breakdown of their storage form, glycogen, in muscle — are the predominant source of moment-by-moment fuel during adequate food consumption. Lipids, in contrast, are a source of metabolic and structural chemicals and either an immediate source or storage form of fuel.

Lipids, as opposed to either proteins or carbohydrates, are of primary concern in governing the amount of body fat stored. Some scientific studies have proved that weight loss can occur by allowing normal intakes of all foods while lowering intakes of only lipids.[4] (See Chapter 42.)

A wide range of interrelated biochemical systems controls whether foods are used for immediate fuel or stored as glycogen or fats. However, when excess food is consumed beyond that required for energy demands, stimulating the ongoing release of insulin, the pressure is to convert this food to storage forms of fuel...primarily as deposited fat.

Lipids manufactured in the liver or absorbed from the digestive tract are transported as very low density lipoproteins (VLDL) and chylomicrons. These sacs, if you will, with membranes permit the transport of lipids throughout a body made up predominantly of water. (See Appendix II.) If it were not for these amazing emulsifying structures, our bodies would separate into oil and water phases like a vinegar and oil salad dressing.

At the adipose cell membrane, the enzyme lipoprotein lipase (particularly efficient in some obese people) breaks down the triglycerides within the VLDLs. Triglycerides are reduced to glycerol, which is transported back to the liver, and fatty acids which, within the adipose cell, combine with glycerol 3-phosphate derived from blood sugar to then form storage triglycerides. If there is high blood sugar, (common with high refined starch and sugar diets), high VLDLs and insulin (usual in the obese), the result will be deposition and accumulation of lipids within the swelling adipose cell.

High blood sugar, VLDLs and insulin stimulate fat deposition

Stored fat is not a static blob in the body. It is biochemically dynamic with mechanisms to not only increase its size, but also to decrease it through seversion. The adipose cell can, in reverse, break the triglycerides that have been stored down to release free fatty acids bound to albumin into the blood stream to provide fuel. This latter process occurs when blood sugar levels and insulin levels are low. This is all complex biochemistry which reduces simply to one principle: Eat sweet, fat and confectionary type foods, and reap the body fat (see Figure III-1).

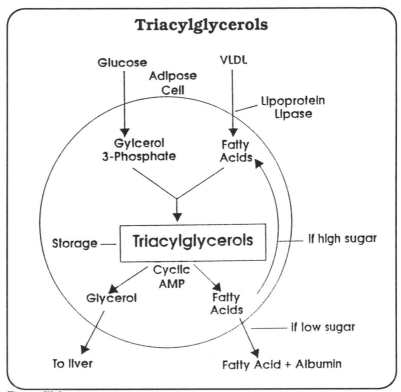

Triacylglycerols

Figure III-1

Lipid
deposition
can
establish
a pattern
of "normal"
above
a healthy
weight

During the course of a year there are fluxes in food consumption, energy demands, and weight. This is normal. Weight maintenance mechanisms are capable of keeping an organism homeostatically in a healthy weight range if unusual stresses are not applied to it. But these mechanisms are exceedingly complex and involve a multitude of hormone messengers, feedback mechanisms, enzymes, transport mechanisms, oxidation cycles, and so forth. A disruption of any one part, like the weakening of a link in a chain, can jeopardize the integrity of the whole. Such is our synorgonic world.

A sedentary lifestyle, the consumption of excess calories — particularly of the concentrated kind found in modern-day foods — excesses of dietary fat, exclusive consumption of pancreatic draining processed foods, and perhaps a wide range of other environmental stresses can challenge adaptive and homeostatic mechanisms and result in ex-

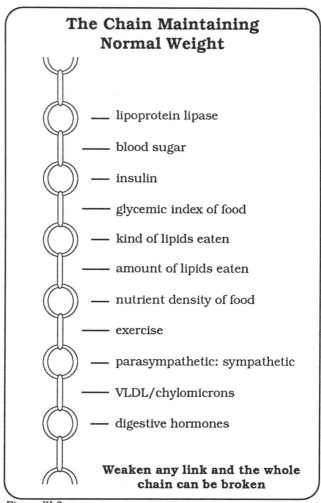

The Chain Maintaining Normal Weight

— lipoprotein lipase

— blood sugar

— insulin

— glycemic index of food

— kind of lipids eaten

— amount of lipids eaten

— nutrient density of food

— exercise

— parasympathetic: sympathetic

— VLDL/chylomicrons

— digestive hormones

Weaken any link and the whole chain can be broken

Figure III-2

Weight must be reversed by solutions that address complexity

cessive weight accumulation. Patterns can be set in terms of increased size and number of adipose cells and excessive stimulation of hormones and other regulatory compounds, which signal the deposition of storage fuels. Such patterns can make the fat deposition process more efficient and make reestablishment of normalcy exceedingly difficult.

Weight control is therefore best addressed on a preventive basis. This is not to say that after an abnormal weight has been established that all is lost. It does mean, however, that the solution is a return to normal homeostatic mechanisms. Quick fixes that deny the complexity of the biological system do not create long-term success. The need is to restore the holistic organism to a healthy, self-regulating and adjusted state.

---

1. Sjostrom, L. "Fat cells and body weight" in *Obesity.* Philadelphia: W.B. Saunders Co., 1980.
2. Ibid.
3. Pi-Sunyer and F. Xavier. "Obesity" in *Modern Nutrition in Health and Disease.* Philadelphia: Lea & Febiger, 1988, p. 797.
4. Hofmann, A.F. and Mekhigian, H.S. "Bile acids and the intestinal absorption of fat and electrolytes in health and disease" in *The Bile Acids*, Vol. 2, New York: Plenum Press, 1973.

APPENDIX IV - COMPANION ANIMAL RECOMMENDATIONS

The principles of the Synorgon Diet apply as well to companion animals as they do to humans.

Herbivores (horses, llamas, goats, cows, etc.) should have access to fresh, natural forage. If supplemental foods are given, these should be designed to preserve the whole and natural character of the food.

Companion animals are victims of human error

Companion dogs and cats are more susceptible to the lifestyle and dietary vagaries of their owners than the larger herbivores, which at least usually have access to fresh pasture. Cats and dogs often live their entire lives eating nothing but what is supplied to them from a bag or a can.

Determining whether a pet is obese is somewhat subjective. Usually increased fat can be felt over the ribs, in the thorax area, on the back, around the pelvic area, and over the abdomen. In the dog, for example, fat will also accumulate over the vertebral and pelvic points at the base of the tail and over the sternum. The ribs should be faintly discernible by the human eye and easily palpable in a normal-weight animal. But weight normally accumulates slowly and it is often difficult for an owner to discern an animal's weight problem until it becomes advanced.

248

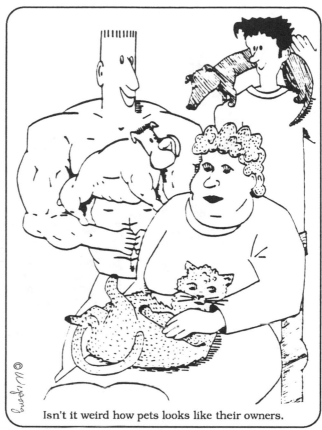

Isn't it weird how pets looks like their owners.

Figure IV-1

For animal owners, a trip to a veterinarian and an evaluation may be necessary to get an objective analysis.[1]

A 100 percent complete manufactured diet is logically absurd

Exclusive processed pet food feeding has been entrenched by the veterinary, academic, and nutritional communities, who permit claims on labels such as, "contains 100 percent complete and balanced nutrition." We have all been lulled by bloated advertising dollars into believing convenience, fun, and health come out of packages. The

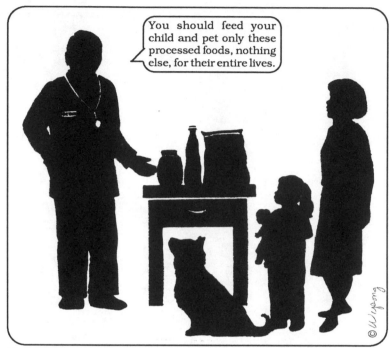

You should feed your child and pet only these processed foods, nothing else, for their entire lives.

Figure IV-2

claim that a fractionated, synthetically forti-fied, processed food can provide "100 per-cent" nutrition is logically absurd. It has, and will, result in a variety of health compro-mises.

Recent evidence, for example, has proved this claim to be inappropriate. The evidence has linked deficiencies in zinc, taurine, po-tassium, and carnitine to diets that were labeled "100 percent complete and balanced" and were even putatively highly researched through feeding trials. (For more details see page 263, no. 6.)

A wave of special formulas has been re-cently produced to curtail weight gain and cause weight loss in pet animals. These diets are restricted somewhat in calories and usually contain high levels of filler fiber materials. Attempting to treat obesity with a single nutrient like fiber is like humans attempting to reduce by eating only grapefruit (see Chapter 15). Treating imbalance by imbalance is fraught with potential dangers. High levels of fiber, which would never be found in the natural diet of a carnivore, potentially can complex and deplete a variety of nutrients, including critical minerals. Food fraction-based, additive laden, synthetically fortified, fiber diluted, modern pet food does not recognize the complex nature of obesity. This commercial approach will not result in long-term weight normalcy, and it may very well predispose to malnutrition and poor health.

Fiber does not solve obesity

Although companion animals (dogs and cats) in the wild would consume some fiber by grazing and eating the vegetation-filled viscera of their prey, high levels of concentrated fiber from such ingredients as peanut hulls, oat hulls, or beet pulp would never be a steady fare as they are in some commercial animal reducing diets. The use of high levels of fiber in companion animal foods must be considered highly experimental, because natural carnivores would never consume such quantities in a wild setting.

Commercial anti-obesity diets may compromise health

However, processed cat and dog diets are extremely convenient and unlikely to be replaced by the natural food of carnivores — live prey. Nevertheless, their diet can be significantly enhanced by home preparation of grocery store primary foods, including fresh meats and organs and properly prepared fruits, vegetables, and grains. The principles of preparing these foods would be the same as for preparing human meals.

Properly prepared home foods provide superior pet nutrition

The shorter digestive tract of carnivores does not permit complete microbial digestion of plant carbohydrates, as is possible in the extended lengths of intestines and multiple fermentative stomachs of cows and other herbivores. Consequently, grains need to be cooked (or ideally, germinated) to properly inactivate antinutritional factors and to gelatinize starches so they will be available for digestive breakdown. Many fruits and vegetables can be eaten raw and are often desired by these species. Most carnivores in the wild will graze on vegetation and consume the fermented, vegetation-filled viscera of their herbivorous prey. Clean meats and organs can be eaten raw or lightly cooked.

An $8 billion pet food industry obscures truth and health

Given in variety, this fresh, whole food diet will be balanced and will provide close to the same anti-obesity features as the natural synorgonic wild diet. (For further help in home preparation of pet foods, see pages 260, 261 and 263, no. 6.)

Sometimes the obvious gets obscured when the obvious means change. Processed pet foods are a significant industry — about $8 billion per annum. Such size creates many vested interests in industry and even in supposedly neutral corners, such as academia and government, which can be

Pet food ingredients are inferior to grocery store ingredients

subsidized by industry in one way or another. Recently, in a debate with a nutritionist, the challenge was made to me that there was no evidence that natural homemade meals had any merit over modern processed cat and dog foods. I countered with the argument that this could not be true unless there is some unidentified special magic that happens to ingredients after they pass through extruders, pellet mills, or retorters (common processing machinery for animal foods). An animal owner can purchase whole grains, fresh fruits and vegetables, and meats and organs directly from the grocery store and feed them to companion animals. On the other hand, the ingredients used in many processed animal foods are often made of food fractions (soy mill run, brewer's rice, middlings, and discards of the meat industry, such as chicken heads, feet, and viscera). These fractions are then subjected to high temperatures and pressures which can further vitiate any nutritional value. It is diffi-

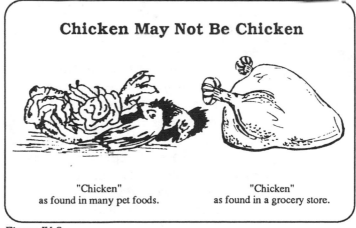

Chicken May Not Be Chicken

"Chicken" as found in many pet foods.

"Chicken" as found in a grocery store.

Figure IV-3

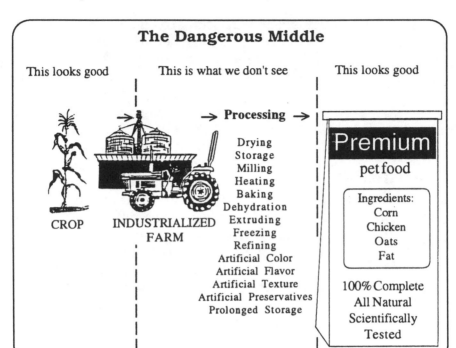

Figure IV-4

cult to imagine how these products can then somehow achieve merit over the original whole fresh item, even if they are so-called "fortified" with a variety of synthetic amino acids, vitamins, and mineral preparations.

Short-term survival does not equal optimal nutrition

Because animals are known to survive eating such modern processed foods, this is taken as proof, by many, that these diets are complete. But simple survival is not the goal of life. Similarly, extending the amount of time a person can survive in a critical care unit or a nursing home should not be the goal of modern medicine. The goal should be optimal health. Eating whole, fresh, natural foods, as close to their natural form as pos-

*Manufac-
turers of
pet foods
must be
carefully
scrutinized
for their
health
motives*

sible, offers many nutritional and health benefits — including the maintenance of normal weight. Given regularly, simple, fresh, raw bones (chicken wings, necks, beef knuckles, etc.) do much to prevent the present epidemic of tooth and gum disease in pets fed processed goop for a lifetime. They also help the pet expend incredible energy, prevent boredom, and eliminate constant begging.

But, as stated above, processed diets are here to stay. When they are used, they should be carefully chosen. The principles we have discussed throughout this book apply. Is a diet designed primarily to enhance optimal nutritional value, or is it designed to

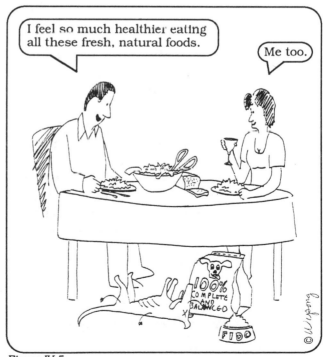

Figure IV-5

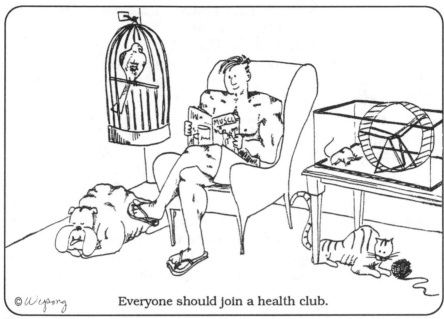

Everyone should join a health club.

Figure IV-6

be simply economical, highly palatable, aesthetically pleasing, and reflective of the current nutritional guess work as to what "100 percent complete" nutrition actually is? A good processed food must incorporate ingredients which are naturally high in nutritional value. It must be processed in a way that enhances nutrition while decreasing the potential damage from the processing. It must be free of non-nutrient additives; stabilized to protect fragile nutrients; and packaged, stored, and delivered by methods that provide as much freshness as possible. Even when such processed foods are used, it is still advisable to alternate or mix these with fresh, natural, home-prepared meals as often as possible.

These principles, when applied to companion animal nutrition along with other outdoor lifestyle modifications, such as lots of opportunity for outdoor exercise, can do much to protect and augment the health of animals. With that will come, without even directly addressing it, normal weight.

---

1. MacEwen, Gregory, VMD. "Fat Cats and Dogs." Petfood Industry, Watt Publishing 31 (July-August 1989): 30.

MORE RESOURCES BY DR. WYSONG

Human and Environmental Health

ED057 *The Wysong Review,* ed. Dr. R. L. Wysong. Arguably the best monthly health newsletter there is. Designed to stimulate thought and action to make a better future. Also explores current research on personal, planetary, and social health. Dozens of current scientific publications are reviewed to provide up-to-date information relevant to medicine, nutrition, ecology and many other important health-related topics. An excellent way to keep up-to-date monthly, and always have fresh provocative ideas to ponder and incorporate into a meaningful life. A yearly subscription (12 issues) is $69.95. Individual newsletters are $6.00. Special introductory bonus packages are available for new subscribers. Request information.

EDC77 *Empowerment,* Dr. R. L. Wysong. A 60-minute audiocassette. Explains the philosophic basis for the Wysong approach to health, nutrition, social problems and the environment. Knowledge is power and with the provocative, inspiring information in this tape you need no longer to be a pawn of commercial interests or a victim of the "experts." Starts you on the road to controlling your own health destiny. $14.95.

ED001 *Rationale for Nutrition,* Dr. R. L. Wysong. A strong, thought-provoking essay justifying the superiority of natural foods and the need to judge technology on its foresight, its understanding of long-term health, and its justice for future generations. 36 pages, booklet, $5.00.

ED101 *101 Things You Can Do To Save Your Life... And The World Too While You're At It,* Dr. R. L. Wysong. (Fall 1993) 101 chapters devoted entirely to helping you optimize your life and our world. 101 examples of simple things that you can do to better take care of your body and your environment. This book is a thought-provoking, educational, and humorous guide to exercise, eating, environmentalism, and much more. Filled with specific resources. 220+ illustrated pp; softcover, $12.95.

ED085 *The Synorgon Diet: Achieving Healthy Weight In A World Of Excess*, Dr. R. L. Wysong. A fresh look at the underlying causes of obesity in modern society. No fad diet or magic exercise, but rather a rationale for life-long changes which can restore normalcy to weight and protect against the wide range of obesity-related diseases. Approximately 270 pages; softcover, $12.95.

ED050 *Lipid Nutrition: Understanding fats and oils in health and disease,* Dr. R. L. Wysong. An A to Z overview of lipids (fats and oils) in human and animal nutrition. Dr.Wysong focuses on new findings which demonstrate that fats are not just carriers of calories, but dynamic nutritional biochemicals that can affect health in profound ways. How the modern processed diet has perverted lipid nutrition to lay the basis for a wide range of degenerative conditions is discussed in detail. Specific recommendations are discussed to improve fatty acid nutrition. Complemented with dozens of excellent drawings and diagrams. 170 pp. referenced; softcover, $12.95; hardcover, $14.95.

ED022 *The Creation-Evolution Controversy,* Dr. R. L. Wysong. A provocative study of the subject of origins. Scientific point-counterpoints are delivered in a highly educational, even-handed, and even entertaining fashion. This is an eye-opening, mind-expanding literary work of great assistance in understanding the limits of human knowledge. Widely read internationally and used as required reading in many college classes. In its 9th printing. 455 pages, scientifically referenced; softcover, $9.95; hardcover, $15.95.

Animal Health

EDV84 *Video: "Rationale for Animal Nutrition — An Interview with Dr. R. L. Wysong."* This video is excellent for personal, educational or group showings. A 70-minute program with two 35-minute, graphically augmented segments, it is stimulating, controversial, and thought-provoking. Discussion encompasses why commercial so-called "100% complete and balanced" foods are not only a myth but a danger; how to cut through pet food marketing hype; what the optimal diet is for your pet; many principles to increase the health of people also; and much more. Definitely a "must-see" and "repeat-see" for anyone concerned about better health for themselves, their pets, or even the Earth. $19.95.

ED800 *Book: Rationale For Animal Nutrition,* Dr. R.L. Wysong. This educational text was produced to be used as a companion to the "Rationale for Animal Nutrition" video or as a stand-alone text to be used for careful study of Dr. Wysong's nutritional and health concepts. The text follows the video and contains many of the charts, diagrams, and photos used in the 70-minute video. $9.95.

ED067 *The Myth of The "100% Complete" Diet,* Dr. R. L. Wysong. A polemic against the claim that manufactured diets using modern processing methods, food fractions, and synthetic vitamins and minerals can be complete and balanced. The "100% complete" claim commonly used in animal foods to build consumer confidence is shown to serve vested interests in the food industry rather than the nutritional well-being of consumers. A revealing exposé with compelling logic. Shakes the very underpinnings of a basic nutritional tenet. Also included is correspondence with journal reviewers who had rejected the article for publication. Presents interesting insight into biases present in the scientific review process. 40 pp, booklet, $5.00.

ED900 *Pet Health Alert,* Important new information revealing why pets are increasingly suffering from heart disease, arthritis, dental disease, diabetes, cancer, auto-immunities, food allergies, obesity and a host of skin, coat, eye, ear, and digestive afflictions. This special report can arm you with the knowledge necessary to keep your pet from being a victim. $4.00.

ED901 *Fresh and Whole,* Dr. R. L. Wysong. An informative brochure designed to help pet owners get involved with their pet's diet. Interesting and educational insights concerning many topics such as: What Is Food?, Fresh Means Raw, Whole Is Best, and Why the Sum of Some of the Parts Does Not Equal the Whole. The brochure also includes simple recipes for specific health conditions as well as answers to some "old wives tales." 32 pp, $2.50.

ED002 *Thought for Food,* Dr. R. L. Wysong. A series of articles published in journals describing the merits of "nutrition first," more natural foods. Various challenges are made to the traditional food processing approaches, and options for improving the food supply and thus optimizing health are discussed. Thought provoking and highly informative to both professional and layperson. 13 pp, pamphlet, referenced; $2.50.

ORDER FORM

BOOKS

❑ ED050 Lipid Nutrition: Understanding fats and oils in health and disease (soft and hard cover) $12.95/14.95

❑ ED085 The Synorgon Diet: How To Achieve Healthy Weight In A World Of Excess $12.95

❑ ED800 Rationale for Animal Nutrition $9.95

❑ ED101 101 Things You Can Do To Save Your Life - And The Rest Of The World, Too, While You're At It (Winter - 1993) $12.95

❑ ED022 The Creation - Evolution Controversy (soft and hard cover) $9.95/15.95

NEWSLETTERS

❑ ED057 The Wysong Review $69.95

BOOKLETS

❑ ED900 Pet Health Alert $4.00

❑ ED901 Fresh and Whole $2.50

❑ ED001 Rationale For Nutrition $5.00

❑ ED067 The Myth Of The "100% Complete" Diet $5.00

❑ ED002 Thought For Food $2.50

VIDEO/AUDIO TAPES

❑ EDV84 "Rationale For Animal Nutrition" (video) $19.95

❑ EDC77 "Empowerment" (audio tape) $14.95

Sub Total _____

Shipping (Free, if order over $10) $2.00

Total [   ]

FREE CATALOGS
Select 2 Free
Additional Choices are $1 each

❑ 1. Wysong Library — A catalog of over 200 Books, Tapes, and Videos.

❑ 2. *The Wysong Review* — A monthly newsletter empowering people with fresh ideas and current research on personal, planetary, and social health.   Special introductory subscription information and catalog of back issues.

❑ 3. The Wysong Healthy Alternative Store — A catalog of over 1000 products available by mail order. Special Co-op Program entitles members to 20% discounts off foods, appliances, personal care and environmental products.

❑ 4. Warning — Before You Take Another Vitamin Read This — A brochure describing vitamin myths and product solutions.

❑ 5. Healthy Personal Care Products Catalog — Biologically compatible products which feed the skin with natural nutrients.

❑ 6. Companion Animal Diets and Supplements.

❑ 7. Equine Nutritional Products.

❑ 8. Wysong Logo Clothing Catalog — A selection of sportswear using the beautiful Wysong Logo.

Total Amount Remitted $_____
(2 are free, $1.00 for each additional)

Mail to:
Wysong
1880 North Eastman Road
Midland, Michigan 48640

263

INDEX

Symbols

276 miles   23

A

A vitamin is a vitamin   144
Absorption   61
  inhibitors   163
Acarbose   163
Activity, Low   137
Addiction   75, 89
Addictive
  fractionated foods   148
Adipose (fat) cells
  number of   242
Adipose cell
  increased number of   137
  increased size of   137
  size of   242
Adipose cells   10
Adipose tissue   242
Adoptees   70
Affluent malnutrition   148
Age
  basal metabolic rate
  decreases   107
Agriculture   32
Air
  fresh   220
Alcohol   79
Alpha-glucosidase
  inhibitor   163
Alphabet   141
Amino acids   134
Amphetamine   93
Amphetamines   79, 163
Anorexia   21, 109
  nervosa   39, 82
Anorexic drugs   92
Anthropometric   48

Antioxidants
  A, C, E   193
  synthetic   158
AO-128   163
Appetite   96
  for high-fat foods   127
  suppressants   163
Arginine   215
Arthritis   38, 132
Atelectasis   166
Atheromatous plague   160
Atherosclerosis   38, 144, 158
Attitude   119
Autoimmunity   132
Autonomic nervous system   76

B

Badminton   110
Balloons   165
Barley and wheat grass
  juice   193, 204
Behavioral modification   118
Beta cells   133
Beta endorphins   84
Bile   237
Biliary stasis   168
Biochemical individuality   71
Blood sugar   244
Blue-green algae   193, 204
Bomb calorimeter   59, 102
Brain   64
Brain stem   96
Bread   141
Broccoli   144
Bulimia   21, 39, 82, 109
Butorphanol tartrate   84
Butter   206

C

Caffeine   163
Caloric intake   179

264

Calorie 57
Calorie is not a calorie 60
Calories
  carbohydrate 59
  protein 59
Cancer 39, 111
Candy 143
Canola oil 206
Capillaries 40
Capitalists 221
Carbohydrate
  refined binges 92
Carbohydrates
  emphasize complex 198
  refined processed 91
Cardiovascular disease 111
Carnitine 215
  acyltransferase 67
Carnivore 98
Carnivores 252
Carotenoids 145
Cat foods 144
Cats 12, 248
Cattle 105
Cell membranes 153
Cereals
  whole grain, cooked 193
Change
  rate of 3
  resistance to 4
Change should be gradual 177
Charts 48
Check up 109
Chickens
  Greek range 146
Children 17, 137
Chinese 60
Cholecystokinin 96, 112, 237
Cholesterol 52, 238
  oxidized 144, 160
Choline 145, 228
Chromium 216
Chylomicrons 240, 243
Cis- forms 145
Clumsiness 38

Cocaine 79
Coconut oil 206
Cold intolerance 122
Companion animals 12, 119, 248
Companions
  seek healthy 184
Complexity *xvi*, 15, 55
Conjugated 158
Consumers 221
Context
  natural 21
Copper deficiency 143
Cortex 76
Cravings 122
Croissants 143
Crutches 214
Cultures 53

D

Deaths 28
Deception 48
Deep fried foods
  avoid 206
Deficiencies 39
Deficiency 168
  copper 143
  iron 143
  zinc 142
Dehiscence 167
Delayed healing 39
Depression 89, 122
Dermatitis 39
Dermatoses 38
Desaturated 158
Dexedrine 163
Diabetes 38
  mellitus 132
Diet
  one day 218
  fads 44
Diets
  low calorie 151

Digestion 61
  lipid 237
  thermic effect 63
Digestive coaters 163
Diglycerides 238
Dogs 12, 248
Dopamine 77, 93
Double bonds 154
Drugs 214

E

E. T. aliens 27
Earth resources 222
Ease 44
Eat
  take time to 190
  portions and leave some 197
Eicosanoids 52
Electrical
  needs of Boston, etc. 33
Electro-bioimpedance 48
Emotional tolls 41
Endorphin high 109
Endorphins 77
Energy 57
Environment
  disruption 10
  restore the 210
Environmental
  context *xvi*, 22
  ethic *xii*
  toll 29
Enzyme blockers 163
Enzymes 243
Ephedrine 163
Ephedrine/caffeine combina-
    tions 216
Epidemics 71
Epidermal growth factor 70
Esterified 158
Ethanolamine 228
Euphemisms 48
Exercise 61, 102, 185, 221
  salons 44
Experiment 24

Experts 44
Eye-mouth gap 117

F

Factory farming 34
Fastin 163
Fasting 168
Fat
  excess on Americans 33
  soluble vitamins 140
  substitutes 163
  tooth 57
  yearly consumption 143
Fats
  saturated 66, 206
Fatty acid structure 223
Fatty acids
  and cholesterol oxidized 206
  essential 140
  omega -3 66, 168
  omega -6 linoleic 66
  omega -9 oleic 66
  trans- 230
Fenfluramine 93, 163
Fiber 111
  craze 145
  in pet foods 251
  rich foods 198
  supplement 112
Fiduciary responsibility 45
Filter for decision making 220
Fish
  cultured 147
  oil 145
  out of water 26
Flavors
  reduce 200
Flax seed oil 193
Fluid retained 179
Food
  efficiency 127
  excess 137
  junk 20
Foresight 181
Fortified 141

Four food groups   143
Fractionated diet   143
Free-radicals   154
French fries   154
Fruit
  as sweetener   193
  dried   193
  fresh   193
  juice   193

G

Gain and loss   125
Galanin   70, 148
Galen   2
Gallstones   39, 168
Gasoline   33
Gastrointestinal distur-
    bances   111
Gastroplasty   165
Genetic
  roots   20
  time warp   26
Genetics   70
Ginger   214
Glucose   64
  tolerance   39
Glycemic index   95
Glycerol   64, 224, 238
  3-phosphate   244
Glycogen   63, 127, 178
Gout   39
Grains in variety   198
Grapefruit   167
Greek egg yolk   146
Greenhouse gas   33
Guidelines   173

H

Hamburger   32, 144
Healing
  delayed   39
Health
  club   110
  eat for   176

problems   38
spa   103
Hedonists   221
Herbivores   248
Heroin   79
Hibernating   105
Hogs   105
Homeostatic (normal)
    baseline   122
Homeostatic (body) baseline
  new, larger   137
Honesty   50
Hormonal abnormalities   39
Hunger   96
Hydrogenated   158, 161
  oils   206
Hydrostatic procedures   48
Hypercholesterolemia   38
Hyperplastic   107
Hypertension   38
Hypertriglyceridemia   38
Hypertrophic   107
Hypoglycemia   39
Hypothalamus   96

I

Industrial World   23
Information age   6
Inositol   228
Insulin   134
Intelligence   46
  necessary   14
Interventions   162
Iron deficiency   143
Isomerized   158
Isomers   229

J

Jaws
  wired   165
Jejunoileostomy   166
Junk food   20

K

Kelp 204
Krypton 48

L

Label 213
Lean muscle body mass 125
Lecithin 145, 228
Leech 90
Leisure 20
Lifestyle 220
  patterns 220
Limbic primitive core 75
Limit of weight that can be
    lost 126
Linoleic acid 225
Linolenic acid 225
Lipase
  gastric 237
  pancreatic 237
Lipid
  absorption 239
  biochemistry 223
  digestion 237
  nomenclature 225
Lipids 51
  processed, altered 55
Lipoprotein 240
  lipase 127, 244
  very low density 243
Lose without dieting 211
Lupus erythematosus 132

M

Mass
  lean body 106
Meal substitutes 167
  substitute drinks 169
Meals
  number or size 192
  simplify 195
  thermogenic effect of 193
Measuring fat 48

Meat eating
  environmental toll 32
  evidence in support 35
  inefficiency 31
  source of fat 30
Medical errors 4
Medications 214
Membranes 51, 230
  fatty acid composition 182
Menus 220
Metabolic setpoint 168
Methadone 79, 84
Methane 33
Micelle transport 238
Micronutrients
  foods rich in 204
Milk
  formula 202
  rice 193
  soy 193
Minerals
  trace 207
Mirror 50
Mitochondria 67
Modern
  society 27
  world 22
Monoamine oxidase inhibi-
    tors 92
Monoglycerides 238
Mood 89
  swings 134
Morphine 79, 80
Mortality 28
  rate 39
Multiple sclerosis 132
Muscle 106
Music 82
Myasthenia gravis 132

N

Naloxone 82
Narcissistic extremes 106
Natural foods merits 144
Natural World 23

Nature 21
Negative feedback 80
Neurological development 140
Neuropeptide (brain chemical)
    imbalance 70
Neurotransmitter gratifica-
    tion 119
Nicotine 79, 163
"No preservatives" trend 158
No-Doze 216
Noradrenalin 93
Nursing 202
Nutritionists 17
Nutrition
    100 percent compete and
        balanced 249
Nuts
    soaked, chopped, raw 193

O

Obesity
    android 10
    defined 10
    economics 11
    gynoid 10
    hyperophic 10
    hyperplastic 10
    incidence 11
    morbid 10
Obetrol 163
Obstetrical 39
Olive oil 206
Omega -3 53, 160
    fatty acids 168
    fish oils 146
    natural sources of 208
Omega -6 160
Omega -9 53, 161
On and off switch 98
Opioid agonists 84
Opportunists 221
Over consumption and under
    nutrition 148
Oxidation 154
Oxygen 154

P

Packaged foods
    if low in fat 205
Pain centers 75
Pain reflex 44
Palm oil 206
Pancreas 133
Parasympathetic 76, 107, 183
Pavlovian pleasure 84
Pellagra 142
Personality 115
Pet foods
    industry 252
Pharmacologic agents 162
Phaseolamin 163
Phentermine 163
Phenylpropanolamine 93
Philosophy
    required 1
Phospholipids 140, 228, 238
Pica 97
Pima Indians 71
Pizza 143
Play 221
Pleasure centers 75
Pneumonia 166
Pollen 204
Polluting the body 222
Polycythemia 39
Polymerized 158
Pondimin 163
Popcorn 167
    air-popped 194
Potatoes 141
Preadipocytes 242
Pregnancy 97, 202
Prevention 45
Pro-biotic powder 193
Processed foods 24
Processing 111, 142
    food 154
Processors 60
Profiteering dangers 14
Protein sparing modified
    fast 169

Proteins
    three-dimensional struc-
      ture 145
Psychological 105
    disorders 39
"Pull" theory 115
Purslane 146
"Push" theory 115

R

Rate of weight loss 179
Rats 61
RDA
    people don't meet 147
Recidivism rate 129
Recipe 220
    books adapted 220
Reductionism 59
Resting metabolic functions 61
Rice 142
Ruminants 33
Running 221

S

Satiety 96, 112
Saturated fats 66, 206
Scurvy 142
Secretin 237
Sentient 35
Serine 228
Serotonin 89, 134
Set-point 107
Single food type diets 97
Skin-fold calipers 48
Snacks
    baked, oil-free 194
Snoring 39
Sodium-to-potassium ra-
    tio 147
Sodium/potassium pump 61
Soft drinks 143
Spirulina 193, 204
Sprouts 198
Starvation 29, 126, 168

Sterility 38
Strenuous 103
Stress 39, 71
Sudafed 216
Sugar 143
Sun 221
Sunflower oils 206
Supplements
    enzyme 193
    mineral 193
    percent who take 148
    vitamin 193
Surgery
    increased risk 39
Surgical interventions 164
Sweet tooth 57
Sympathetic 76, 107, 183
Synergy 7
Synorgon
    defined 9
Synorgonic fiduciary responsi-
    bility 221
Synthetic sweeteners 163

T

Taurine 144
Technology
    dangers 13
Teflon® 165
Thermic loss 61
Thermogenesis 61, 70
    enhancers 163
Thinness 221
    genes 70
Thromboembolism 167
Thyroid 70
    hormones 133
Time
    & Adaptation 23
    required 122
Timeline 23
Tolerance 39, 97
Too much of too little 141, 148
Toxicities 39

Trans-
  form 145
  isomers 161
Transport 61
Treadmill 109
Triglyceride 224
  fluidity 233
Triglycerides
  long-chain 66, 161
  medium-chain 67, 161
Tryptophan 91, 134, 215
Twins 70

U

Unsaturated essential fatty
    acids 154

V

Vaccinations 133
Vagus nerve 165
Varicose veins 38
Variety 195
Vegetables 194
Very low calorie diets 168
Very low density lipopro-
    teins 243
Vitamin
  A 140
  C, natural 144
  D 140
  E 140
  K 140
Vitamins 207

W

Waist-to-hip ratio 127
Walking 221
Water supply 33
Weight level
  difficulty in resetting body to
      lower 137
Weight lifters 187
Whole, fresh, raw, foods 202

Whole, raw foods 66
Wild 72
  animals 12
  game meat 146
  setting 65
Work 221
Wound infection 167

X

Xenon 48

Y

Yogurt 193
Yo-yo cycles 125
Young 137

Z

Zinc deficiency 142